DEVELOPMENT IN ADOLESCENCE
Psychological, Social and Biological Aspects

DEVELOPMENT IN ADOLESCENCE

Psychological, Social and Biological Aspects

W. EVERARD
Institute of Clinical Psychology
University of Utrecht

C. B. HINDLEY
Institute of Education
University of London

A. BOT & J. J. van der WERFF ten BOSCH
Institute of Physiology
Erasmus University of Rotterdam

1983 **MARTINUS NIJHOFF PUBLISHERS**
a member of the KLUWER ACADEMIC PUBLISHERS GROUP
BOSTON / THE HAGUE / DORDRECHT / LANCASTER

Distributors

for the United States and Canada: Kluwer Boston, Inc., 190 Old Derby Street, Hingham, MA 02043, USA
for all other countries: Kluwer Academic Publishers Group, Distribution Center, P.O.Box 322, 3300 AH Dordrecht, The Netherlands

Library of Congress Cataloging in Publication Data

Main entry under title:

Development in adolescence.

Based on a postgraduate course for medical practitioners, held in Leiden, Nov. 1981, which was entitled, Adolescence: psychological, social, and biological aspects.
1. Adolescent psychology--Addresses, essays, lectures. 2. Adolescence--Physiological aspects--Addresses, essays, lectures. 3. Adolescence--Social aspects--Addresses, essays, lectures. 4. Adolescent psychopathology--Addresses, essays, lectures. I. Everaerd, W. [DNLM: 1. Adolescence--Congresses. 2. Adolescent psychology--Congresses. 3. Human development--Congresses. WS 460 D489 1981]
BF724.D45 1983 155.5 83-8051
ISBN 0-89838-581-4

ISBN 0-89838-581-4

Copyright

PRINTED IN THE NETHERLANDS

PREFACE

Depending on the definition of this concept that is adopted, adolescence is the narrow threshold or a vast no-man's land that separates adulthood from childhood. In one -physicalist- view, adolescence begins when secondary sex characters become noticeable and ends when they are fully developed. In another -sociological- view, adolescence ends when social independence has been gained. It may easily take many years more to span the interval between those two events.

In this collection of papers by specialists from various disciplines, physical, psychological and social aspects of adolescence are considered.

The book originates from a postgraduate course for medical practitioners, who deal with adolescents, but the range of the papers is such that we hope it may be of value to a much wider readership, including educators and all who are concerned with adolescents. The course was entitled: 'Adolescence: psychological, social and biological aspects', and was held in Leiden in November 1981. It was the fourth in a series of Boerhaave Courses instigated by the Dutch Growth Foundation of which a published record has now become available. Previous titles are 'Somatic growth of the child' (1966), 'De samenstelling van het menselijk lichaam' (1968) (=Human body composition), and 'Normal and abnormal development of brain and behaviour' (1971).

The detailed programme of the course was planned by Dr. F.J. Bekker, Prof. Dr. J.L. van den Brande, Prof. Dr. W. Everaerd, Prof. A.Th. Schweizer and Prof. Dr. J.J. van der Werff ten Bosch.

It is a pleasure to acknowledge the skilful technical support given during the preparation of this text by Mr. H. van Beek of the Department of Automatic Signal Processing, Erasmus University of Rotterdam.

THE EDITORS

CONTENTS

CONTRIBUTORS

A.A.J. Bartels — Paedologisch Instituut
1075 AZ Amsterdam
The Netherlands

Lea Dasberg — Pedagogisch Didactisch Instituut
University of Amsterdam
1015 DT Amsterdam
The Netherlands

R.F.W. Diekstra — Institute of Clinical Psychology
University of Leiden
2312 KM Leiden
The Netherlands

W. Everaerd — Institute of Clinical Psychology
and Psychotherapy
University of Utrecht
3512 JK Utrecht
The Netherlands

C.B. Hindley — Department of Child Development
and Educational Psychology
University of London Institute
of Education
London WC1H OAA
U.K.

D.J. de Levita — Department of Child Psychiatry
University of Amsterdam
1105 BC Amsterdam
The Netherlands

June Machover Reinisch — A.C. Kinsey Institute for
Research in Sex, Gender and
Reproduction
Indiana University
Bloomington, Indiana 47401
U.S.A.

J.W. van Seters | Institute of Social Education, University of Utrecht, 3508 CC Utrecht, The Netherlands

G. Sinnema | University Children's Hospital, University of Utrecht, 3512 LK Utrecht, The Netherlands

N.W. Slot | Paedologisch Instituut, 1075 AZ Amsterdam, The Netherlands

C.J. Straver | Netherlands' Institute for Social and Sexuological Research, 3704 EB Zeist, The Netherlands

F. Wafelbakker | Chief Medical Office of Health, 2265 BA Leidschendam, The Netherlands

J.J. van der Werff ten Bosch | Institute of Physiology, Erasmus University of Rotterdam, 3000 DR Rotterdam, The Netherlands

J. de Wit | Paedologisch Instituut, 1071 AK Amsterdam, The Netherlands

P.H. Wolff | The Children's Hospital Medical Center, Boston, Mass. 02115, U.S.A.

1. A HISTORICAL AND TRANSCULTURAL VIEW OF ADOLESCENCE

LEA DASBERG

If history can be of any use to the field of education it is so by destroying some illusions. First of all the illusion that human life can once and for all be divided into neatly limited periods, like infancy, childhood, adolescence, adulthood, old age. Secondly that all these periods can be exactly defined and determined within unchangeable time-limits: being the same for the Egyptians of the Old Empire as for the Dutch people of the postindustrial era; for today's inhabitants of a city like New York as for the members of an isolated African tribe; or the same for the working class as for the bourgeoisie. Such unchangeable lines of demarcation do not exist. The time-limits of infancy or of adolescence change from one historical period to another, from one culture to another and from one social class to another. In the third place the word 'transcultural' should not arouse expectations that I will refer to Eskimoes and Maoris. I am a historian, not an anthropologist. Culture for me means lifestyle, and transcultural means differences of lifestyles, not so much between ethnic groups as between historical eras and social classes within the western world.

At one moment in time adolescents can consist of: boys and girls in school or boys and girls working in a factory; boys and girls writing poems in a diary, or fighting for a guerilla group; boys and girls experiencing the initial rites of their tribe into manhood and womanhood, as well as boys and girls undergoing a lonely and guilt-ridden experience of masturbation. At the same time, even within the same culture and in the same social class, there are adolescents still wondering what cohabitation is like, while others have already experienced abortion.

These contrasts do not imply that adolescence does not exist. It does, but explicitly in western society. One definition at least is possible: adolescence is the stage of life between childhood and adulthood. So what <u>is</u> childhood and what <u>is</u> adulthood? I would define childhood as existing as long as a person is taken care of within protective surroundings. There are some exceptions: soldiers in the army, monks and nuns in convents, old people in homes, and delinquents in prison. I would define adulthood as starting from the moment a person definitively leaves the protective environment and has to take care of himself. In other words: a person reaches adulthood from the moment he bears social responsibility.

Besides social responsibility we also know juridical and political responsibility, but we will not take that into account because juridical responsibility commonly follows some years after a person has assumed social responsibility, and because the general right to vote is a very recent phenomenon. Before its acceptance by democratic parliaments even the oldest and wisest men were politically children.

So a child lives within a protective environment that is responsible for him. An adult has left this protection and is responsible for himself. An adolescent stands on the threshold of these two situations.

Another common illusion is that adolescence is a universal phenomenon. It is, however, a <u>cultural phenomenon</u> typical of modern western societies like ours. Anthropological studies like Margaret Mead's COMING OF AGE IN SAMOA (1) showed that in that culture adolescence is almost non-existent. There is only a quantitative difference between childhood and adulthood, not a qualitative one. So there is no place for a threshold implied by the term 'adolescence'. From a very young age the child takes part in such adult activities as fishing, hunting, woodcutting, defence against wild animals, human enemies and the natural elements. Thus the child does not have to leave a protective environment nor explore an absolutely different kind of life after the age of 12 or 14, and quite abruptly transfer responsibility from his parents' shoulders on to his own. The transition from childhood to adulthood in such cultures is nearly invisible.

In cultures where adolescence came into existence it is limited to particular social classes. In our society it started as a phenomenon of the middle-class and aristocracy. For children of artisans and craftsmen in pre-industrial times, and after the Industrial Revolution for proletarian and peasants' children, adolescence did not exist for centuries.

In the 16th and 17th centuries, in western society, boys and girls of the 12 to 16 years age group who belonged to these lower social classes were normally full-time labourers. The artisan boy was taught to help in his father's workshop from his 6th or 7th year on, and at the age of 11 or 12 was sent away from home to undergo his apprenticeship under the guidance of a master. He then bore responsibility for the quality of the workshop's products. As an apprentice he wandered from one master to the next till he was recognized as a master himself. During these wandering years the lad was about 14 to 18 years old. Although he slept and ate in the household of his masters he had himself to organize his next destination, his travelling, his clothes and his earnings. He bore his own social responsibility. He did not show any resemblance to our present teenager or adolescent (2).

As far as a girl of that time and social class was concerned the position was similar. She also started working with her mother from the age of 6 to 7 years. Household work in those days easily took 14 hours a day. It was not uncommon for the mother to give birth once a year, so that daughters between 10 and 15 years old had to take over the full responsibility of cooking, washing, mending the clothes, educating the younger children, feeding the babies, doing the shoppings, milking the cow, bargaining with the merchants, and so on. The possibility of losing her mother in childbirth and of being burdened with the full responsibilities of the household was far from theoretical. Like the boy of those times the girl did not have much in common with the teenager or adolescent girl of our days. There was virtually no visible threshold between her girlhood and her own marital life and motherhood (3).

Middle class boys and girls in the 17th, 18th and 19th centuries sometimes left their own lessons at school, or from a private tutor, at the age of 15 to immediately become a private tutor themselves for other children under other people's roofs. A Dutch example is Justus van Effen. Thus in their life too there was no transitional period between childhood and adulthood (4).

So adolescence is not only a cultural phenomenon, and a phenomenon of social class, but also a <u>phenomenon created by history</u>.

However, there is one aspect of adolescence that is inevitably common to all cultures, all social classes and all historical eras, namely, adolescence as a biological phenomenon. The bourgeois child and the proletarian child, the western and the oriental child, the medieval and the child of today, are all, at a certain moment in their development, confronted with the physical changes of puberty resulting in sexual maturity.

But we have to be careful not to confuse adolescence only with this process of growing towards sexual maturity. We have to put the question what kind of consequences this sexual maturity brings forward for the boy or girl in question, if any at all! We can think of lots of consequences. The consequence for prince William II of Orange and the girl Mary Stuart in the 17th century was their marrying at the ages of 13 and 11 years, and not only as a formality for dynastic purposes. Directly after the wedding ceremony, the meal and the festivities, the royal and noble guests accompanied bride and bridegroom to their marital bed to be present for their first intercourse, and to give directions and advice (5). The consequences for Neeltje Doff, a working class girl from the slums of 19th century Amsterdam, were that her parents forced her to sell her nearly mature body as a prostitute as soon as possible, in order to feed her starving little brothers and sisters (6,7). The consequences for a girl of the same age in the same city, but living in one of the splendid merchants' mansions at one of the 'grachten', were that her mother or her nanny, moved to tears, told her that now she was a big girl and that later on she would learn to understand what that meant. When this girl herself became a mother of a daughter of 14, she tried to help her by giving her a booklet about the bees and the flowers, because she remembered how awfully frightened she was at the sight of the first menstrual blood without having any explanation (8).

Only in the last of these three stories was there evidence of an adolescence as we understand it, a life period between childhood and adulthood, involving shock and curiosity, pride and shame, longings, and fear concerning the fulfilment of these longings, and both alienation from and a new consciousness of, one's own existence. In the life of the noble couple and of the proletarian prostitute there was no time between childhood and adulthood for such a period of curious and fearful exploration into the world of adults.

Returning to our 17th century lad wandering as an apprentice from one town to the other, we did not call him an adolescent because he was already responsible for his own living. However, though <u>socially</u> living an adult life, was he perhaps <u>sexually</u> an adolescent in our modern sense? In a poem of Karel van Mander (1548-1606) this poet-painter advises these boys -and he himself had been a boy like them- in the following way: to become a capable artisan, he says, you have to work hard and to learn a lot. But sometimes Cupid and Bacchus and their son Hymen will distract your attention so that you will do bad work and your master will be angry. You are not allowed to marry until you have become a master yourself. But that does not mean that you cannot start to explore, and take a little snack from time to time. Complete abstinence will cause you headaches and bad moods. Marry when you are 25, but you must have already discovered the secrets of marriage by then. For girls it is different. Although for them too there should not be a long interval between reaching maturity and experiencing sexual intercourse, they should have their experiences within the bonds of marriage. So the ideal couple for a wedding is a man of 25 and a girl of 17 (9,10,11).

In this picture of his time which Karel van Mander sketches for us, a kind of adolescence had come into existence, as far as boys were concerned, but only in part. A socially independent young man had to postpone a regular sex life and marriage until he could be economically responsible for a whole family.

From another source we know about third grade pupils of Latin school at the end of the Middle Ages, boys of about 11 years old, being publicly punished before all the pupils and the staff of their school for having visited lupanaria (brothels) (12). Here we have an early example of adolescence as we have known it since Victorian times, a position of absolute social dependence on parents and teachers, closely supervised, but already conscious of new passions and feelings and searching for a release from them, in a society that requires the postponement of such experiences until social independence is reached.

Kant (1725-1804) saw the moment youngsters acquired the ability to be parents themselves as the end of education and of youth, and consequently as the end of guarding and protecting them. He thought an age of about 16 was appropriate (13). His contemporary Rousseau did not agree at all. For him there had to be an interposed period of exploration of the adult world which should take place between the 20th and 25th years (14). But even this had to be in the charge of an adult guide, who would not allow these explorations to extend beyond the borders of the mind! For years and years a boy and a girl in love with each other had to explore each other's minds by reading books together, by visiting each other under a chaperone's eye, and had to examine the purity and truth of their love by leaving each other for long periods of travelling the world to become mature and wise enough for ... yes, for sexual intercourse, but immediately within the bonds of marriage!

The higher the social class of the child, the longer its adolescence lasted, socially, economically and biologically, because the growing wealth, especially after the Industrial Revolution, equipped more and more parents with the means to give their children a prolonged education under expensive and careful guidance. The youngsters were banished to the nursery with their nanny or private tutor, in order not to hear the adult conversation in the salon. They were kept away from the mother in childbirth and even from the cat giving birth to its kittens. From before the awakening of maturity, boys and girls were segregated in separate boys' and girls' schools. Books with information about human biological and physical processes were locked away from them. Instead they were stuffed with false information about childbirth by the intervention of the stork or the cabbage. Girls were taught to sleep with their hands outside the sheets, without understanding why. Boys were forced into anti-masturbation belts (8, pp. 207-211). Rousseau's propaganda for a child's own exploration of the world; its own observations of nature itself rather than learning from books; his emphasis on the need for sensory experiences of cold and warmth, wet and dry, colour and scent, excluded the exploration and observation of one's own body, one's own genitals, one's own secretions, let alone that of others! He and his fellow educators blocked these areas of exploration by clothes, sheets, and above all by taboos. If a child's nature was stronger than the prohibitions and it sought and found satisfaction underneath the bedclothes, his lust was overpowered and overshadowed by guilt. Perhaps the adolescent could still find his body secretly, but he did not dare to love it. Even if he obtained some knowledge of sexuality, his feelings and experiences remained virginal. Rousseau's theory that the lad should not have his first sexual intercourse before the age of 25 became daily reality in the upper classes. And when he finally entered this realm he was scared to death. It might take another five years for his sexual activities to reveal something of lust and joy, if it ever happened.

Imagine these healthy teenagers from the upper classes in the time between 1750 and 1940, how, crying bitter tears into their pillows and clenching their fists in despair, they longed for the angel with the flaming sword to come and expel them from Rousseau's Paradise of Children's Innocence, and to chase them to the grim planet of sin, lust, responsibility and self realization (15). Among the lower social classes, adolescence did not become such a torture. There the children could observe the bodies of their brothers and sisters sleeping in the same bed with them; were not banished from the mother in labour; and knew that their unmarried sister became fat because she was pregnant. How radically sexual behaviour changed in moving from one social class to another we learn from an autobiography of a 19th century factory labourer Willy Bromme. Born of lower middle-class parents, he fell into a proletarian mode of life by bad fortune. After some years of protected education in Latin School, suddenly at the age of 12 he had to enter the factory as a common labourer. At the sight of the factory girls stripped naked to change into their working outfit, he was deeply shocked and ashamed, and turned his eyes away. He despised his fellow workmen for not only looking at the naked girls' bodies, but also for touching them. He also held the girls in contempt for not only permitting such advances, but shamelessly inviting them and enjoying them. As a result of increasing poverty his parents had to let some rooms of their house to boarders and the innocent boy was confronted with the nightly visitors of these new inhabitants of his home, even lesbian ones. How swiftly then this virginal lad from Latin School changed into a grown-up male with an adult sex life. Finally he was obliged to marry very young because his girl was pregnant (16). This true story is like a spontaneous laboratory experiment proving that two absolutely different kinds of adolescence could exist in one and the same person within a very short time, as a result of the transition from the social class of Latin School pupil to the social class of factory labourer.

The laws prohibiting child labour along with compulsory school education for everybody brought into existence a new kind of youngster, intellectually much more skilled and mature than people of their age in former centuries, but economically and socially much more childish than their great-grandfathers had been at their age. At the end of the 19th century for this new kind of boys and girls, a third educational milieu, in addition to the first (the family) and the second (the school), was needed and created: the youth movement. In this environment the adolescent could practise his intellectual skills as a president of the club meetings or as a club treasurer; he could expend his suppressed energies in long marches as a scout; he could translate his longings for political heroism into loud community singing around the camp-fire, or at the ceremony of the swearing allegiance to the flag; and he could sublimate his awakening physical passions by erotic feelings for a bosom-friend, or for an idolated youth leader or teacher (17-22).

Better medical care, improved dietary rules, gymnastics as an obligatory part of the school curriculum, increased possibilities for sport, all caused an acceleration of the development of the body. So in the last 50 years the first menstruation in a girl's life advanced from the age of 14 or 15 to the age of 11 or 12 (23,24). This physical acceleration produced a psychological refusal to postpone all kinds of experiences (25). Children took jobs during school vacations to earn their own money; began to have sexual intercourse shortly after reaching biological maturity; and participated in political activities, no longer within a youth movement guided by adult leaders, but within the real political arena of demonstrations. Their right to vote was advanced by several years in most countries, in our own from the age of 21 to the age of 18.

We can follow these changes in adolescence by reading teenagers' diaries from about 1900 till now. Charlotte Buehler was the first one to use boys' and girls' diaries as a scientific source (27-29). In the girls' diaries she published from the time of the First World War, and in the boys' diaries from the twenties, political themes are absent, with the exception of <u>one</u> passage about a train full of soldiers leaving for the battlefield and a Red Cross vacation colony for half-starved children of the big cities. The young writers are not only not conscious of the political situation, and that in a country at war, Austria, but equally of belonging to a certain social class, or of the very existence of social classes at all, again with the one exception of the same girl who noticed the war. Almost totally absent are sexuality, sexual feelings, and sexual longings. Only one of the girls' diaries records a crush on a female teacher, evidently a sublimation of her erotic feelings for the woman. Only one boy student of a 'Gymnasium' writes about his raving for a girl he is not allowed to meet or to speak to, except at dancing school: 'Never, never will I be allowed to offer all my treasures to a girl, because -you know- we are not allowed to love really without marrying ... oh, perhaps, once, once, to love stormily and with all my intensity ... but no ... three steps backwards please - or marriage!' (28, pp. 94-95).

We get quite a different picture from boys' and girls' diaries between 1939 and 1953. Their age varies from 12 to 18, their social class from the Austrian 'Gymnasium' to the factory. The diaries were collected by the leader of their youth movement, the Reverend Wolfgang Fischer (15). Especially the boys' diaries are very frank about sexuality by this time. They are full of self accusations for the sin of masturbation, and the boys shed hot tears caused by their feelings of guilt. They despise themselves for the deed they describe as filthy and beastly. Their youth leader does not see it as his duty to help them to get rid of their guilty feelings. On the contrary, when one of the boys succeeds in sublimating these passions into an erotic veneration for his 'Fuehrer', for instance, by following him slavishly, his leader cheers this as a moral victory to be proud of (18).

What about diaries of adolescents nowadays? In 1953 Muchow (30) came to the conlusion that writing diaries had become increasingly rare, so that a psychology of youth based on diaries would certainly give us a totally distorted picture of youth nowadays. He is convinced that sexual intercourse as a quite normal practice in the daily life of young adolescents today, absorbs sexual fantasies and longings that before had to be sublimated into erotic and spiritual emotions, and that these pent-up emotions had been one of the important reasons for writing diaries.

Nevertheless, today's early sexual experiences do not bring back the pre-Victorian situation of an abrupt transition from childhood to adulthood, without an intermezzo of adolescence - on the contrary. Of all the characteristics of adulthood the youngsters have only won some sexual freedom, while they have not obtained economic independence, juridical and financial accountability, or political rights, in short: social responsibility. They still are not adults. But they are not children either. Their situation is that of the intermezzo called adolescence.

Adolescence, instead of disappearing lasts longer and longer. The reasons for this lie partly in such conditions of our society as prolonged schooling and unemployment, but also, in part, because the path to adulthood became blocked to young people by their own disapproval of the adult world. They have not been taught to take serious decisions. They are afraid to devote themselves to a profession they value because of the economic instability. They fear marriage because of today's frequency of divorces (31). They condemn procreation because of overpopulation (32). Their attitude is an escape of responsibility, a fear of freedom as Fromm called it (33). Of course this does not apply to all of them, probably not even a majority, but nevertheless quite a number.

Instead of the vanished youth movement this fear of freedom brought new kinds of juvenile subcultures into being, offering the possibility of hiding in a group, conforming to its codes, obeying its rituals, of belonging to a clan of equals (34,35). These subcultural groups vary from innocent disco-clubs to dangerous hell's angels, from playful punks to desperate junks. Sometimes, instead of the erotic veneration for a youth leader this fear of freedom brought them to follow blindly a guru or a mystic sect (36,37). And for those who are too individualistic to look for the protection of a group, the fear of freedom, the fear of responsibility more and more often ends in juvenile suicide (38-42).

Adolescence has often been romanticized as the most promising time in man's life. I think we have to regret that we ever let it assume such proportions. It has become a torture that we must help adolescents to overcome as soon as possible.

REFERENCES

1. Mead M. 1959; first edition 1928. Coming of age in Samoa. A psychological study of primitive youth for Western Civilisation. New York:William Morrow.
2. Emmerich W. 1974. Proletarische Lebenslaufe. Autobiografische Dokumente zur Entstehung der Zweiten Kultur in Deutschland. Band I: Anfaenge bis 1914. Reinback bei Hamburg: Rowohlt.
3. Power E. n.d.; first edition 1924. Medieval people. New York: Doubleday (Anchor Books), pp. 99-125.
4. Heyboer-Barbas ME. 1956. Een nieuwe visie op de jeugd uit vroeger eeuwen. Een letterkundige studie ter vergelijking van het Nederlandse kind vroeger en nu. Nijkerk: Callenbach, p. 21.
5. Kernkamp GW. 1943. Prins Willem II. Amsterdam: van Kampen (Patriareeks), Ch. 2.
6. Doff N. 1970. Dagen van honger en ellende. Amsterdam: Meulenhoff.
7. Doff N. 1973. Keetje Tippel. Amsterdam: Meulenhoff.
8. van Ussel JMW. 1969. Geschiedenis van het sexuele probleem. Meppel: Boom.
9. Hoecker R (ed). 1916. Den grondt der edel vrij schilder-const. In: Das Lehrdicht des Karel v. Mander. Den Haag: Martinus Nijhoff, verse 1,1; 1,61; 1,63.
10. De verscheyden lessen Petri Messiae, Edelman van Sivilien, Tot Leyden, By Jan Claeszoon van Dorp, woonende inde vergulde Sonne, 1595.
11. Miedema H. 1973. Karel van Mander, Den grondt der edel vrij schilder-const, vol. II. Utrecht: Haentjes Dekker & Gumpert.
12. Post RR. 1954. Scholen en onderwijs in Nederland gedurende de middeleeuwen. Utrecht/Antwerpen: Het Spectrum, p. 128.
13. Langeveld MJ. 1959. Bijdragen tot het gesprek van systeem en historie in de opvoedkunde. Acta Paedagogica Ultrajectina 19, 58.
14. Rousseau JJ. 1762. Emile ou de l'éducation. Edition used: Classiques Larousse, livre 5.
15. Fischer W. 1955. Neue Tagebuecher von Jugendlichen. Die Vorpubertaet anhand literarischer Selbstzeugnisse. Freiburg i.Br.: Hambertus. Grundfragen der Paedagogik 2.
16. Bromme MThW. 1971; photomech. reprint of the first edition 1905. Lebensgeschichte eines modernen Fabriksarbeiters. Frankfurt a.M.: Athenaeum.
17. Blueher H. 1916. Wandervogel, Geschichte einer Jugendbewegung. Prien: Kampmann & Schnabel.
18. Blueher H. 1918. Die Deutsche Wandervogelbewegung als erotisches Phaenomen. Prien: Anthropos.
19. Seidelmann K (ed). 1966. Die Deutsche Jugendbewegung. Bad Heilbrunn: Klinkhardt (Klinkhardt's Paedagogische Quellentexte).
20. Seewann G. 1971. Oesterreichische Jugendbewegung 1900-1938, 2 volumes. Frankfurt a.M.: Dipa.

21. Harmsen G. 1961. Blauwe en rode jeugd. Ontstaan, ontwikkeling en teruggang van de Nederlandse jeugdbeweging tussen 1853 en 1940. Assen: van Gorcum.
22. van der Louw A. 1974. Rood als je hart. 'n Geschiedenis van de A.J.C. Amsterdam: Arbeiderspers.
23. Langeveld MJ. 1972. Groeien, leiden, kiezen. Enige aspecten van de persoonlijkheid in zijn ontwikkeling tot volwassenen. In: Europa 2000. Perspectieven voor een aanvaardbare toekomst. Deventer: Kluwer.
24. Bullough VL. 1981. Age at menarche: a misunderstanding. Science 213, pp. 365-366 (relativates this opinion but not quite convincing).
25. Soentgerath A. 1967. Paedagogik und Dichtung. Das Kind in der Literatur des 20. Jahrhunderts. Stuttgart/Berlin/Cologne/ Mayence: Kohlhammer, p. 33.
26. Huelsenbeck CJ, Louman J, Oskamp A. 1970. Het rode boekje voor scholieren. Utrecht/Antwerpen: Bruna.
27. Buehler Ch. 1927. Zwei Maedchentagebuecher. Quellen und Studien zur Jugendkunde 1, 2nd edition. Jena: Fischer.
28. Buehler Ch. 1925. Zwei Knabentagebuecher. Quellen und Studien zur Jugendkunde 3, with an introduction on Die Bedeutung des Tagebuchs fuer die Jugendpsychologie. Jena: Fischer.
29. Buehler Ch. 1934. Drei Generationen im Jugendtagebuch. Quellen und Studien zer Jugendkunde 11. Jena: Fischer.
30. Muchow HH. 1953. Jugend im Wandel. Verlag Hildegard Bernaerts, p. 14.
31. Lockhorn E. 1980. En wat gebeurt er dan met mij? Kinderen over echtscheiding. Baarn: In Den Toren (Anthosboek).
32. Kluvers I, Veenhoven R. 1980. Kinderen - ja of nee? Ervaringen, opvattingen en achtergronden. Baarn: In Den Toren (Anthosboek).
33. Fromm E. 1970. Escape from freedom. New York: Avon (Discus Books).
34. Roszak Th. 1969. The making of a counter culture. Reflections on the Technocratic Society and its youthful opposition. New York: Doubleday (Anchor Books).
35. Simmons JL, Winograd B. 1968. It's happening. A portrait of the youth scene today. Santa Barbara, California: Marc-Laird (with a list of the group's own vocabulary!).
36. Koellen K. 1980. Jeugdsecten in Nederland. Amsterdam: Allert de Lange.
37. On the sect of the People's Temple of the pseudo-priest Jim Jones, Haagse Post, Dec. 2, 1978, nr. 48, pp. 6-9
38. de Graaf AC, Diekstra RFW. 1980. Opnemingen in algemene ziekenhuizen wegens suicidepogingen in de periode 1970-1976. Nederlands Tijdschrift voor Geneeskunde 124, 149-153.
39. On the observations of Dr. J. Weinberg of the psychiatric center 'Het Curium', Oegstgeest: Kinderzelfmoord. Haagse Post, Dec. 23, 1978, nr. 51/52, pp. 44-51.
40. Proceedings 7th International conference for suicide prevention, Amsterdam, August 27-30, 1973, Speyer N, Diekstra RFW, van de Loo KJM (eds). Especially pp. 142-156 (Diekstra), pp. 158-159 (Kamaras).

41. Schuelerselbstmorde. 1980. Betrifft Erziehung 13 (4), 21-31.
42. Diekstra RFW, Koster A, van der Leeden B. 1980. Kinderen en zelfmoord. Ouders van nu, april.

FURTHER LITERATURE

Bakan D. 1971. Adolescence in America: from idea to social fact. In: Daedalus. Boston: American Academy of Arts and Sciences, pp. 979-995.
Beets N. 1954. De grote jongen. Utrecht: Bijleveld.
Bondy C. 1956. Pubertaet als sozialkulturelles phaenomen. In: Moderne Entwicklunspsychologie. Berlin: Luttke, pp. 89-96.
Coleman JS. 1967. The adolescent society: the social life of the teenage and its impact on education. New York/London: The Free Press of Glencoe.
Demos J, Demos V. 1969. Adolescence in historical perspective. Journal of Marriage and Family 31, 632-638.
Flitner A, Hornstein W. 1964. Kindheit und Jugendalter in geschichtlicher Betrachtung. Zeitschrift fuer Paedagogik 10, 311-339.
Friedenberg E. 1962. The vanishing adolescent. New York: Dell Laurel.
Garland E. 1963. The changing face of childhood. London: Hutchinson.
Hornstein W, Flitner A. 1965. Neue Literatur zur Geschichte des Kindes- und Jugendalters. Zeitschrift fuer Paedagogik 11, pp. 66-85.
Hornstein W. 1965. Vom 'Jungen Herrn' zum 'Hoffnungsvollen Juengling'. Wandlungen des Jugendlebens im 18. Jahrhundert. Heidelberg: Quelle & Meyer.
Muchow HH. 1964. Jugendgenerationen im Wandel der Zeit. Vienna: Brueder Hollinek.

2. CONCEPTS OF ADOLESCENCE; THEIR APPLICABILITY TO NORMAL AND CLINICAL SAMPLES

D.J. DE LEVITA

When Oedipus, still ignorant of the role he was to play in 20th century psychology, solved the riddle of the Sphinx, which was, as you know, about a creature that goes on four, two and three legs respectively, he lost another chance of immortality in not mentioning adolescence that could very well have been introduced as a stage of human life where one has no leg to stand on at all. The different names for this stage have varied through history. Before the Second World War 'puberty' and 'adolescence' were two different stages in development in Dutch terminology, adolescence coming after puberty and meaning young adulthood. After the war we have mainly adopted Anglo-American terms, i.e. puberty referring to physical changes and especially secondary sexual characteristics, and adolescence mainly referring to the concomitant psychical changes, or as a broader term, to include all the processes connected with these changes, physical, psychic and sociocultural. Thus in Dutch 'puberteit' and 'adolescentie' are synonyms, the latter having driven out almost completely the first.

Adolescence as a psychological concept was introduced by Stanley Hall. In 1904 he finished a voluminous, encyclopaedic work, 'ADOLESCENCE: ITS PSYCHOLOGY AND ITS RELATIONS TO PHYSIOLOGY, ANTHROPOLOGY, SOCIOLOGY, SEX, CRIME, RELIGION AND EDUCATION' (1). First of all it contains a description of adolescence as a period which reveals enormous possibilities of growth, and encompasses a variety of contradictions such as hyperactivity and lassitude, happiness and depression, egotism and self-abasement, selfishness and altruism, gregariousness and shyness, sensitivity and cruelty, radicalism and conservatism.

The adolescent, involved in so many conflicts, was bound to experience 'storm and stress', i.e. 'Sturm und Drang', a characteristic of adolescence that Hall brought home from Germany where he studied many years before he returned to the U.S. and became a professor at Johns Hopkins. The concept of 'storm and stress' has ever since played an important part in discussions on adolescence, under the heading 'adolescent turmoil', as we shall see later. There is still another idea in Hall's work that is of interest for later conceptualizations. As a Darwinist he was convinced that man in his individual development recapitulated the development mankind had gone through in the course of the centuries, and that this was valid also for mental development. Adolescence, he thought, was to be compared with the period in which mankind had taken its greatest swing and the adolescent was therefore potentially destined for great developmental leaps. As we shall see, this idea of adolescence as the recapitulation of past stages returns unexpectedly in the psychodynamic theory of adolescence.

This theory starts with Freud, who in 1905 in the 'THREE ESSAYS ON SEXUALITY' (2) devoted one of them to what he called the 'transformations of puberty'. Before touching on this issue, however, a few words must be said on the innovations psychodynamic theory implied, compared with the descriptive psychologies. In psychodynamic theory the stages of development were viewed as logically linked to each other by some basic concepts of which they were the successive manifestations in time. These manifestations in their turn were to be viewed as the interactions between the child and his direct environment. In 1905, Freud made the point that many of the passionate, impulsive, emotional swings of adolescence might be, in fact, the corollaries of maturing sexuality, and that they had not come to attention solely on account of the taboos of the Victorian age. Sexuality and aggression became the main forces in this theory, and the infantile forms, especially of sexuality, the determinants of the stages of psychic development.

I want to make two points: 1) about the environment: it was conceptualized mainly in its functions of stimulating or inhibiting the instinctual wishes of the child, and, 2) the only factual, biological substratum available to psychodynamic theory was twofold: the genital distinction between man and woman, and the reproductive capacity in man and woman after the maturation of the reproductive organs in puberty. It is therefore not surprising that the psychodynamic interpretation of adolescence should have had great force and a great ability to renew itself in the course of time.

A theory in which successive stages are viewed as the ever more mature, fuller and richer manifestations of the same basic forces, and cognitive and emotional capabilities, is particularly well fitted to account for psychopathology. The model of the explanations is in fact astonishingly close to biochemical models, in which chains of products, one developing out of the other through the cooperation of all kinds of agents from the outside world, can be arrested or interfered with if the required agents are absent or impaired in quality. The chain can then come to a standstill and pathological products spread throughout the organism. As in biochemistry, the problem in the psychodynamic equivalent of such developmental theory is that there is not one chain of products, but an ever-increasing number of such chains. The first was sexuality which, since it is based on biological facts, still serves to elucidate the main phenomena of adolescence. Other developmental lines added themselves to it: aggression, perception, thinking, regulating mechanisms, individuation, self-esteem etc.

When it becomes more and more complicated, a theory needs some simplification in order to be practically useful, especially when it is to be used widely. Its great simplifier was Erik Erikson (3). He started from the old stages of development, named after the specific precursors of genital sexuality (the oral, anal and phallic phases), but extended their meaning in a way that was on the one hand superficial and reductive, but on the other hand provided an inspired and masterly survey of the innumerable developmental processes which had come to light in observation and psychotherapeutic treatment of children, adolescents, and adults. In his conceptualization of psychic development, the first year of life is characterized by the child receiving whatever care and offers of stimulation are available to him, resulting in the acquisition of basic trust. The major emphasis in this concept is already on the mother, it is: '...first of all a task for maternal care', and works 'by that kind of administration which in its quality combines sensitive care of the baby's individual needs and a firm sense of personal trustworthiness within the trusted frame-work of their culture's life style' (3, p. 221).

Here is one of the roots of Erikson's immense popularity: in one brilliant concept he has united the forces of instinct psychology, the interactions with the environment, in this case the mother, and has opened a window towards a broader, sociocultural conceptualization, in which, through the family as a representative of the current culture or subculture, all influences on the child are modified or, at least, coloured.

Equally, in his version of Freud's anal stage, it is the domination of bowel movement that, together with the acquisition of locomotion and speech, lays the basis for autonomy and independence. Since mastery of bowel movement is identical with having the choice to hold and to let go, these attitudes become fundamental to development but here again Erikson states: 'Culturally speaking, these attitudes are neither good nor bad, their value depends on whether their hostile implications are turned against enemy -or fellow man- or the self' (3, p. 222).

Continuing in this way, Erikson postulates a series of developmental tasks, defined in very general terms, which run all through childhood, until in adolescence a final integration takes place in the form of what he calls 'establishing an identity'. From each of the previous stages and developmental processes a quality is acquired that will grant the adolescent a place in society, a place that he holds in good faith. For each kind of quality that is inherent in this identity, the trace can be followed back to the stage which at its time had to provide the core, the basis for that special quality, such as for instance: optimism that all will go well, from the first year of life; the courage to take initiative and to experiment freely, from the third year of life, etc. The model of development that is presented by the contributions of Erikson and others can be summarized as a kind of steeple-chase, in which the child, with his drives and talents, has to jump over a number of obstacles, put in his way by society, or by his immediate environment as the representative of it, in order to make him adapt to society and, importantly, to what society is likely to have in store for him. If one of the obstacles has been too high, or his capacities in jumping too low, or something unexpected has interfered with his jumping, a refusal may occur or he may have to go on less steadily than he rode before. Then fixations to these developmental tasks that were not performed successfully ensue, so that they may become problems of character, and in that way an inseparable part of the individual. He still has, however, one chance of gaining what he missed during childhood, to compensate for it. That is: adolescence.

Part of the dissent of adolescence can be interpreted as efforts to obtain now what was painfully absent previously, or at long last to take revenge for something one was once too small to fight against. It can mean straightening out something that had been dormant for years, painful, because the parents can be totally unaware of what they did, or failed to do, and the adolescent himself too, generally has no idea about the meaning of his behaviour. Much aggression toward parents is postponed aggression from the time the parents had all the power to impose their will upon the child, and used it in a way they thought best, or in a way that was inevitable to them because of the experiences of their own childhood, or, still more unfortunate, in a way inherent in a fundamental personality disturbance. In these sorts of adolescent behaviour there is always some identification with the parent without the parent noticing it.

> I remember a boy of fifteen who had parents who loved each other dearly, more than they loved their child. Both were intellectuals. They looked after the child properly; he apparently received everything he needed, yet there had always been an almost imperceptible qualitative lack of maternal and paternal love. As if one such loving couple in the house was not enough, there hung on the wall a huge photograph of the Royal Couple of whom the parents, ardent royalists, were very fond. One day, when the parents were on a trip, the boy, who was a talented painter and craftsman, took the photograph down from the wall and out of its frame. With a very small knife he cut hardly visible pieces from the face of the queen and her husband, and put it back on the wall. He described to me how from time to time during the next few weeks, his parents looked at the picture, with perplexity, till his father finally burst out 'what the hell happened to that picture?'

For this concept of adolescence as the conclusion of childhood a basic idea is one that Ernest Jones worked out (4), and that strikingly reminds us of Hall's notion of recapitulation. Jones suggested not that man relives the history of mankind, but that the adolescent recapitulates the early stages of his own development and that the old acquisitions such as being autonomous are now put to the test. This is a more precise way of understanding adolescence as providing a kind of last chance. This view of development is that it constitutes a risky and dangerous journey. It is clear that the model arises out of treatment experiences with children and adolescents, and is one which applies, in the first place, to such treatment.

Loosening the attachments to the parents and family is sometimes a painful process for all the people involved, especially when things that had been highly satisfactory during childhood now lose their appeal without anybody being to blame. All kind of reactions can be found among adolescents and parents to hide feelings of mourning, which for the parents can unfortunately coincide with, or be a part of, a mid-life depressive crisis. Commonly the adolescent, in effect, withdraws his emotional investments from the family and the world of his parents, and attaches himself to his peers who now become his main objects of identification, and his main support in problems. Here there are two points to be made, arising from the investigations undertaken in the sixties about this hypothetical shift from parents to peers by Bowerman and Kinch (5). They concluded firstly that: '... as children become increasingly involved in activities with peers, they become increasingly oriented toward the peer group, particularly with respect to association, and to a lesser extent in accepting the norms and values of the peer group. Second, a lowered orientation to the family during the period of adolescence is not inevitable ... but it is a function of the way in which the family reacts to the child during the period of increasing peer orientation'. In fact it was found that the shift from parents to peers was on the whole much less marked than people had assumed. In their national study Douvan and Adelson (6) state that there are all kinds of big changes, especially in dating, having jobs outside the home etc. but, they say: '...when we look to more subtle and emotional aspects of autonomy, we find changes occurring during adolescence to be more modest. Children, and particularly girls, do not abandon emotional ties to the parents with anything like the ease with which they shift companions' (6, p. 133). Or, to give a few numbers they quote: girls of age 11 spend 22% of their free time with friends and 68% with their family; when they are 18 this is 46% and 44% respectively. Later findings, for instance by Offer and Offer (7) or the Isle of Wight findings of Rutter et al. (8) are in tune with this.

It seems that in healthy adolescents (i.e. in samples of the general population in contrast to clinic patients) the generation gap, and its concomitant conflicts, is much less frequent than was believed. On the other hand it has been confirmed as existing in adolescents who, as children, presented with psychiatric symptoms (9). However, there is a large group in between about which we know nothing: the children who need help but do not get it. As Shepherd et al. (10) have shown, there is a big gap between the need of help and actual referral of a child, and many factors involving the whole family and the personality of the parents have a bearing on it.

So, as regards the issue of 'adolescent turmoil' we are left with the same disagreement as Hall had to face when Thorndike (11) and other outstanding psychologists of his time called his descriptions exaggerated. In a normal sample dramatic scenes or ruptures between parents and adolescents seem to occur only in a minority. In children who presented with psychiatric problems during childhood, an adolescent turmoil may occur, and its absence can even be regarded as a sign of severe psychopathology, as the adolescent may be unable to lessen his attachments to his family. As to inner turmoil, it has been reported by many adolescents who have been investigated, like those in the Isle of Wight study (12) of whom nearly 50% confirmed that they felt misery at times. I wonder, however, what numbers would have been found if adults in the same population had had to answer the same questions. If I may permit myself a personal remark in this respect: the gap between the data collected by empirical investigation and information about the inner life provided by psychotherapists is not one that is to be bridged in the way that Coleman (13) has tried, nor is it a gap that can be bridged. It is a dichotomy that should be accepted as the main characteristics of psychology and psychiatry, respectively.

We now come to the question: if we are thinking in terms of developmental tasks, what is the task of adolescence? All authors agree that the first is: to start love relationships and to integrate sexuality into them. Secondly: to detach oneself from the parental world and to establish one's own identity. For these purposes everything one has gained during childhood is needed: basic trust, autonomy, courage, etc. The first experiences in this direction are very important indeed, and in many respects adolescence can be viewed as the beginning of adult life with many concomitant vulnerabilities and fragilities. Many a distress of adulthood turns out at long last to have its origins not in childhood but in adolescence, and there is a strong need to look there for the ill-remembered but nevertheless significant experiences which hampered adult development and self confidence for a long time. As Michel Sardou (14) expresses it, speaking about love, 'elle fait parfois souffrir tout le long d'une vie'. Not uncommonly, people have amnesias of adolescent experiences not dissimilar to those of early childhood - it must be the feeling of helplessness that makes so many things disappear from memory.

It is of interest here that mechanisms akin to those in adolescence are coming to be seen as operating throughout development in childhood. Mahler (15) described how the nearly one year old, after the symbiosis with mother and the establishment of a truthful relationship with her, uses the safety of their bond as a 'home base' to operate from in exploration of the outside world, comes back to her from time to time for 'refuelling' and then goes out again. Ultimately, some time later, his initial imperviousness changes to frustration, as he misses his mother and starts a movement back to her, an approach in which he returns a sadder and wiser man. The swing from the safe and familiar to the new and unexplored, and then back for new integrations, a feature also to be seen in the work of Piaget (16), seems to be a general developmental principle that we are increasingly observing in many ways.

I would like to make a further point about this. It concerns peers. Traditionally they are expected to emerge during adolescence as the heirs of family life, dropping out of the clear sky exactly as sexuality was supposed to do, a century ago. I think that the significance of peers at earlier ages is underestimated, and that many of the roots of isolation and disturbed relationships with people lie in the nursery school. For many children it is a jungle. The completely new and unique event can occur of meeting somebody who has the same age, and yet at the same time is not connected with them by any family tie. It is often the first person in their life with whom they can lose a relationship as a result of their own behaviour. An important root of the vicissitudes of later love relationships turns out to lie in these first rejections by peers.

All development implies change, and the meaning and importance sociocultural conditions assign to any of its parts may vary. Adolescence, however, seems to be destined to play a major role, whatever the sociocultural conditions under which this role is to be enacted, since it is connected with the biological changes on which the procreation and survival of mankind depend. Erikson (17), viewing it from the summit of the prosperity of the western world, saw it as a moratorium during which adolescents could freely experiment with adult roles before taking on in reality the responsibilities and burdens of adult life, while, obviously, already in possession of many of the privileges adults made adolescents wait for in earlier times.

Bernfeld (18) thought that adolescence was in some way related to artistic creativity, that in some gifted personalities a potentiality for the breaking of existing bonds and the creation of new ones was slumbering, which would bring about a kind of constant and permanent adolescence. Eissler (19) later found this in the life of Goethe and made it one of the themes of his biography of Goethe. According to this concept adolescence is completely detached from its traditional connection with biological development, especially that of the sexual organs, and has been transformed into a purely psychic process which is characterized by the sequence of: attachment-internalization of the bonds into psychic structure-detachment-forming of new attachments.

The shape of adolescence is highly influenced by the place sexuality has in society. Sexuality has long held a key position in the total gamut of privileges our society grants to adults, the more so since it has long been completely forbidden to children. The concept of adolescence as the transition from childhood to adulthood can be seen as a redistribution of privileges and burdens, and adolescence is bound to change in nearly every respect if privileges shift from adulthood to childhood, or if burdens are no longer matched by future prospects. From the still flowing spring of belief in the future, which originated in childhood, adolescents retain their motivation to study, in the face of their growing awareness that they may not be wanted afterwards when they seek a job. The drastic changes we observe in adult society, but also in childhood because some of these adults are parents, will heavily affect adolescence and perhaps will make it disappear again.

REFERENCES

1. Hall GS. 1904. Adolescence: its psychology and its relations to physiology, anthropology, sociology, sex, crime, religion and education. New York: Appleton.
2. Freud S. 1905. The transformations of puberty. In: Three essays on sexuality. In: Standard edition, volume 7. Strachey J (ed). London: Hogarth Press.
3. Erikson E. 1950. Childhood and society. New York: Norton.
4. Jones E. 1922. Some problems of adolescence. British Journal of Psychology 13, 31-47.
5. Bowerman CE, Kinch JW. 1959. Changes in family and peer orientation of children between the fourth and tenth grades. Social Forces 37, 206-211.
6. Douvan E, Adelson J. 1966. The adolescent experience. New York: Wiley.
7. Offer D, Offer JB. 1975. From teenage to young manhood, a psychological study. New York: Basic Books.
8. Rutter M, Graham P, Chadwick OFD, Yule W. 1976. Adolescent turmoil: fact or fiction? Journal of Child Psychology and Psychiatry 17, 35-56.
9. Shepherd M, Oppenheim B, Mitchell S. 1971. Childhood behaviour and mental health. London: University of London Press.
10. Shepherd M, Oppenheim AN, Mitchell S. 1966. Childhood behavior disorders and the child guidance clinic. Journal of Child Psychology and Psychiatry 7, 39-52.
11. Thorndike EL. 1901. Notes on child study. Columbia University Contributions to Philosophy, Psychology and Education 8, 3-4.
12. Rutter M, Tizard J, Whitmore K (eds). (1970). Education, health and behaviour. London: Longmans.
13. Coleman JC. 1978. Current contradictions in adolescent theory. Journal of Youth and Adolescence 7, 1-11.
14. Sardou M. 1973. 'La maladie d'amour' (song).
15. Mahler M. 1975. The psychological birth of the human infant. New York: Basic Books.
16. Piaget J. 1935. La naissance de l'intelligence chez l'enfant. Neuchâtel: Delachauz & Niestlé.
17. Erikson E. 1956. Ego identity and the psychosocial moratorium. In: New perspectives on juvenile delinquency. Washinton DC: U.S. Department of Health, Education and Welfare.
18. Bernfeld S. 1923. Ueber eine typische Form der maennlichen Pubertaet. Imag 9, 169-189.
19. Eissler K. 1963. Goethe. A psychoanalytic study 1775-1786. Detroit: Wayne State University Press.

3. PSYCHOLOGICAL CHANGES IN ADOLESCENCE RELATED TO PHYSICAL CHANGES

C.B. HINDLEY

A clear distinction must be drawn between puberty and adolescence. Puberty refers to the period in which those physiological and anatomical changes occur which transform the child into a physically mature organism, capable of reproduction. Although the times of onset and termination may be difficult to establish with complete accuracy, they are nevertheless reasonably clear (1).

The term adolescence has come to mean something much wider than that of the Latin verb adolescere 'to grow to maturity'. It refers to the entire set of changes in the individual's life occurring between childhood and adulthood, including physical, psychological, and social. There is no very clear time of onset, nor is there a clear time of termination of the process. If having an occupation and being a parent are taken as among the criteria of adulthood in the fullest sense, then a university student would hardly satisfy it, nor would a childless person of 40. This indicates the difficulty of having a clear line of demarcation and, indeed, psychologically speaking, each of us retains childish characteristics only too often in our everyday behaviour. Very broadly, then, we are talking of a period which typically extends from around 10 years to the late teens, or well into the twenties.

Although puberty and adolescence are obviously closely related, a problem can often enough arise from discrepancies between the degree of physical and psychosocial maturity. Thus, a pregnant girl of 15 is certainly physically mature, but neither she, nor the youth who impregnated her, are likely to be psychologically mature enough for parenthood, nor are they likely to be economically independent of their parents.

Historically, the period between birth and adulthood has been divided into several phases from Aristotle onwards, often simply on the basis of age (2, chapter 1). In some tribal societies adolescence hardly occurs, with the child becoming an adult overnight, following an initiation ceremony (3). In Europe, from the time of the ancient Greeks until this century, the vast majority of children have enjoyed no prolonged period of education during the transition from childhood to adulthood, with little in the way of choices, and adolescence as we know it was something that applied only to a privileged few (4).

Turning to adolescence in our own times, perhaps the biggest influence on how we see it was that of Stanley Hall (5). His characterization of it as a period of 'storm and stress' has become part of the folklore of the Western world. That at least this may not be universally true was vividly shown by Mead (6) in her description of adolescence in Samoa as following an easy course. As a result of reviewing varied anthropological evidence, Benedict (7) argued that the extent of 'storm and stress' would depend on the degree of continuity between the role of the child and of the adult in the society in question. Where children were already fully involved in the community's activities, such adolescent turmoil would be absent.

It is to be noted that Hall regarded the developmental processes in adolescence as inherently involving 'storm and stress'. His descriptions were, perhaps, the most graphic expression of the nativist account of adolescent development, but others -such as Gesell- adopted a similar standpoint (8,9). According to these theorists development consists in the unfolding of what is genetically given, with environmental influences exerting at most a secondary role. In complete contrast are the views of social learning theorists such as Bandura (10,11,12), who seek to base their account of development simply on the effects of experience, or learning. Thus turmoil and conflict in adolescence will depend on whether the child's previous development enables him/her to cope with the new demands of adolescence. They did, in fact, find evidence to support this contention, in that adolescents from caring, supportive families, showed much less difficulty than those from rejecting, conflictful homes (11). This point of view is not inconsistent with that of the cultural anthropologists, Mead (6) and Benedict (7), insofar as they -while recognizing the biological changes in adolescence- insist that the role of such changes in the adolescent's development is culturally determined.

Other theorists on the nature of adolescence occupy an intermediate position, accepting that both biological and sociocultural factors play a part. Freud's major emphasis was on a genetically given course of development, but influenced by how the child had progressed through the earlier phases (13,14). How the adolescent would cope with the resurgence of strong sexual instincts after the 'latency' period of childhood, would depend on how the conflicting wishes of early childhood had been resolved. Anna Freud (15,16) has seen what she termed adolescent 'intellectualization' and 'asceticism' as ways of coping with the anxiety aroused by the insistence of the sex drives. Instead of demanding sexual freedom, which can be too anxiety provoking, the demand may be for intellectual or political freedom.

Erikson (17,18) developed Freudian theory further, laying emphasis on adolescence as a crucial period for the individual to discover and come to terms with his/her own identity (who am I?), which involves becoming aware of what he has become, and what he can become. It can therefore be pivotal in orienting the future course of life.

Both Ausubel (3,19) and McCandless (20) see the way in which the biologically given affects the adolescent as being strongly affected by his previous experience with his family and others (8,9). Thus, for McCandless, as with Freud, the adolescent is rather suddenly confronted with his/her sexuality and sex drive, and so has to adapt to it - an adaptation that may involve conflict with previously learnt inhibition of sexuality, in our culture. Unlike Freud, he attaches great importance to the effects of such learning. Sullivan (21) saw inter-personal relationships as of supreme importance throughout life, and therefore the positive or negative attitudes of parents towards an adolescent's sexuality would for him, too, make adjustment easy or difficult.

Mention should be made of Lewin (22), who looked at adolescence in terms of roles. He contended that the childhood role of an ultimate dependency on the parents, and the adult role of independence, were relatively clear and comprehensible. The adolescent role, however, is much more ambiguous, involving features of the other two. An adolescent may be called upon to switch from one to the other at a moment's notice. Thus, parents may expect acceptance of responsibility (adult role) when it suits them, or compliant obedience (childhood role) when that suits them. Internally, the adolescent may experience difficult contradictions between childish wishes to be helped and not to be responsible, and adult wishes to be responsible, to be his own boss. The physical changes, too, may heighten this role conflict, and role confusion. Thus, for Lewin, the extent of stress would depend on the extent of role confusion (8,23).

Several issues arise from this brief review of theories of adolescent development. An obvious one is that the way adolescence is viewed will depend on the general approach adopted to the nature of developmental processes. A second is that the proponents of each theoretical approach are able to offer some evidence to the discovery of which the theory pointed, and which is consistent with the theory. Pragmatically, this suggests that perhaps their accounts are complementary, that each is emhasizing an aspect of what is an extremely complex process. A third point is that while some of the theories -in particular the more biological ones- offer an account which is intended to be universal, it may well be the case not only that adolescence may differ in different societies, but also that there may be substantial individual differences in the process within a society, something which Spranger (24) has claimed (see also 8,25). Offer and Offer (26) have recently found confirmatory evidence for this suggestion from their longitudinal study. They conclude that there are three routes through adolescence, what they term 'continuous growth', 'surgent growth', and 'tumultuous growth'.

As regards the first issue, the nature of developmental processes, I would claim that the day is long past when it made any sense to hold a genetic <u>or</u> environmental view of development. Such an eminent geneticist as Waddington (27,28) has insisted that epigenesis, the process by which the phenotype comes into being from the genotype, always and inevitably involves a dynamic interaction between the hereditarily given and the environment (figure 1). This is true whether we are talking of a cell or of

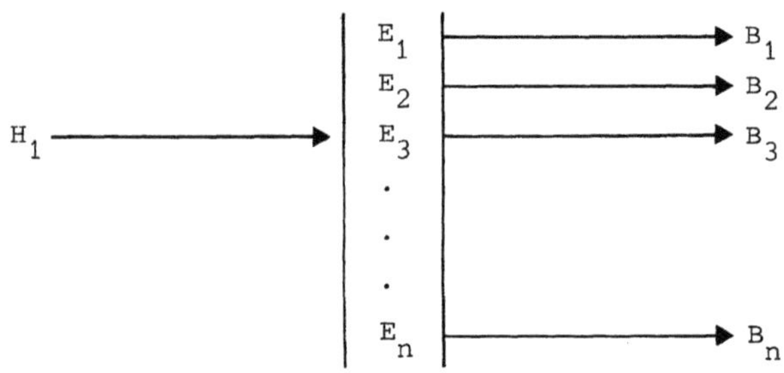

A particular heredity (H_1) in interacting with different environments (E_1 ... E_n) will lead to different behavioural development (B_1 ... B_n).

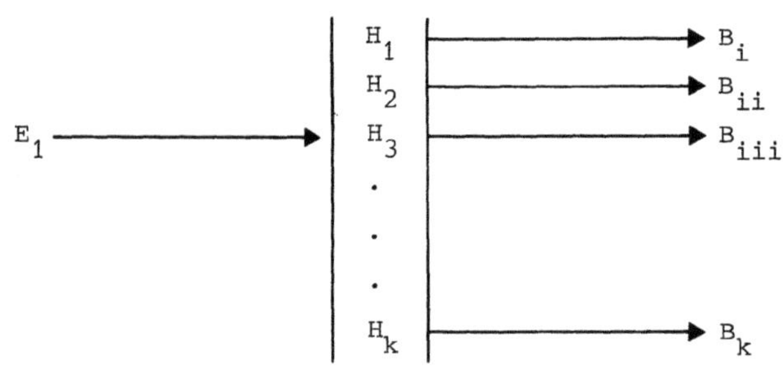

A particular environment (E_1) in interacting with different heredities (H_1 ... H_k) will lead to different behavioural development (B_i ... B_k).

Figure 1. Relationships between hereditary and environmental influences (modified after 9).

a foetus, or whether of physical growth or of psychological development (9,27,28,29,30). Nor does it make any sense to ask for percentage contributions of heredity and environment to development. All development depends 100% on heredity and 100% on environment (9,31,32,33). What does make sense is to investigate the range of variation that heredity produces in interaction with a range of environments (9, chapters 4 and 5).

The implications of this point of view for the study of development in adolescence are: 1) that we are dealing with extremely complex processes, 2) that the elucidation of the functional interrelationships between them is likely to be difficult, and 3) that we should welcome contributions to our understanding coming from any quarter, or from any theoretical position. Also implicit in this review is that not only are there psychological and social consequences of the physiological changes of puberty, but that psychological as well as physical and social environmental factors affect physiological functioning and development (29,34,35,36). Thus, Krech and his colleagues (34) have shown that in rats a stimulating behavioural environment affects the structure and function of the brain.

Leaving aside theories, a very useful analysis which points to the multifarious nature of adolescence is that of Havighurst (37) in terms of the developmental tasks of this period, of which he lists ten. Wall (4) reduces this to four. As he puts it: 'Between 13 and 25, the growing boy or girl has to develop a <u>social self</u>, oriented to others, aware of a place in society, of duties as well as privileges and in general emancipated from dependence on parents or, indeed, on others. A <u>sexual self</u> ... capable of a range of feeling from friendly indifference to deep involvement with a member of the opposite sex, adequate adjustment in marriage and the ability to found and care for a family ... Vocational adjustment, a <u>working self</u>, is also essential not only to economic independence, but as a basis of self-respect and self-knowledge'. This includes 'a certain satisfaction derived from work and of a sense of being needed, and of being something more than a replaceable unit. (Implications in a time of unemployment are obvious - C.B.H.) Finally, however simple it may be, most of us need an interpretation of life, philosophic, religious, political, vaguely or clearly formulated, something by reference to which major decisions can be taken and the behaviour and attitudes of others understood' (4, p. 13).

I will have these developmental tasks in mind reviewing the principal processes going on in adolescence. I will take it for granted that the society we live in sets the scene, and makes its demands, and briefly review the major physical and psychological changes occurring in adolescence, ending with a brief consideration of their interaction.

PUBERTY

The observable features are well known (1). The first detectable signs in boys being the increased size of the testes, followed -a year or so later- by the adolescent growth spurt, and by slight changes in the pubic hair and other secondary sexual characteristics. The duration of the process can vary between two and four years or so (38,39), and ends with the production of live spermatozoa, with the virtual cessation of growth, substantial muscular development, and the other secondary sexual characteristics.

In girls the process begins about two years earlier. Growth of the ovaries is not readily detectable, so the first signs are in the pubic hair, and the appearance of breast-buds. As in boys, there is an adolescent growth spurt. The process more or less ends with menarche, soon after which viable ova are produced, and the secondary sex characteristics are now freely in evidence.

Two interrelated sets of findings in recent years have greatly increased our knowledge of the mechanisms involved (figure 2). One concerns the hormonal feedback system, and the other the role of the central nervous system in controlling the onset of puberty (40,41,42,43). It is now clear that the control of the production of gonadotropic hormones (GTH) by the anterior pituitary lies in the hypothalamus, the medial basal area of which secretes a further hormone -gonadotropin releasing factor (GRF)- which is carried by the hypophyseal portal circulation to the anterior pituitary (44,45). During childhood the amount of pituitary GTH in the blood is small, as any rise in the level of the sex hormones (testosterone, oestrin, progestin) inhibits the hypothalamus from producing GRF. What has been called the hypothalamic 'hormonostat' is then very sensitive. At puberty

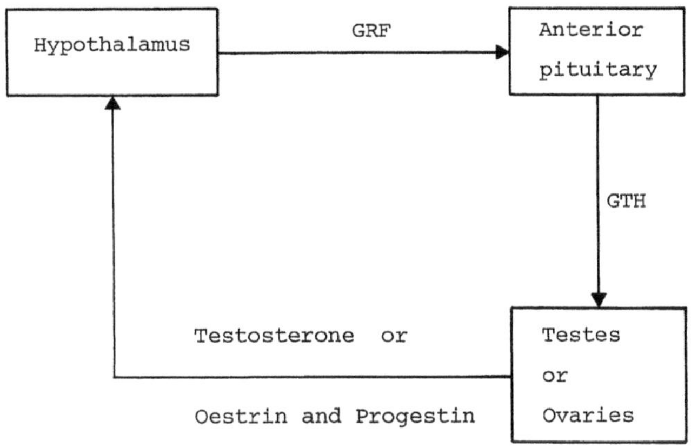

Figure 2. Schematic representation of hormonal feedback system. The medial basal area of the hypothalamus produces gonadotropin releasing factor (GRF) which travels through the hypophyseal portal circulation to reach the anterior pituitary, stimulating production of gonadotropins (GTH). These circulate to the gonads, and stimulate the testes to produce testosterone, or the ovaries to produce oestrin and progestin. These enter the general circulation, effecting the secondary sexual changes of puberty. High concentration of the sex hormones inhibits hypothalamic production of GRF.

the setting of the 'hormonostat' changes, so that production of GRF, and therefore of gonadotropins, is no longer massively inhibited. Large quantities of gonadotropins are produced, and these stimulate the growth of the gonads. They, in turn, produce the sex hormones which are responsible for the major changes of puberty.

What brings about the changed sensitivity of the hypothalamus in humans is not known. As it has wide connections with cortical and other sub-cortical levels of the brain, it is not unreasonable to suppose that various aspects of life experience may affect it. This has certainly been found to be the case in other species in some of which, for example, puberty may be hastened by additional exposure to light, or to minute quantities of chemicals produced by the opposite sex, the pheromones (41,46). Whatever the reason, there is evidence that puberty has been occurring earlier and earlier for over a hundred years in advanced countries at the rate of 4 months per decade (1). Tanner suggests that improved health and diet may be the main factors, but in view of what is being discovered concerning other factors in animals, these may also prove to be of importance in humans.

INTERRELATION OF PHYSICAL, SOCIAL, AND PSYCHOSOCIAL FACTORS

The psychological changes occurring during adolescence are partly a result of the physical changes of puberty, and partly of social influences and demands. Equally, they influence how these physical and social changes are responded to. There is thus a constant interaction between physical, social, and psychological factors (figure 3).

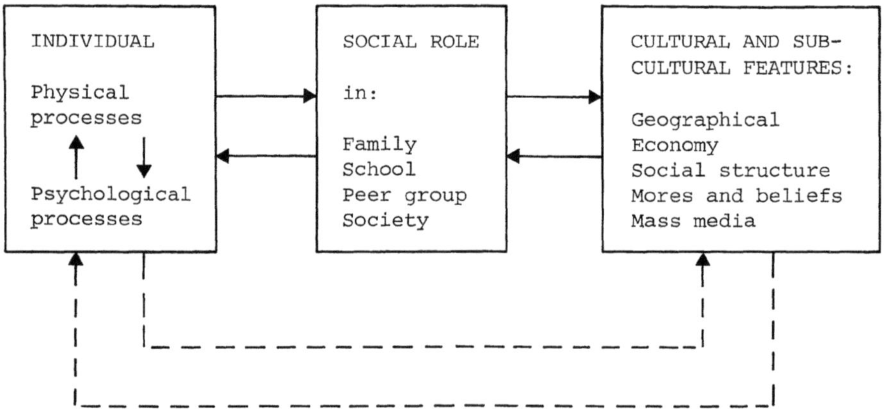

Figure 3. Interrelationships in adolescence. Changes in the adolescent affect his social role and relationships, and are affected in turn by them. Social roles of adolescents are expressed in a culture, and are influenced by it. The culture largely affects the adolescent via the groups in which he participates, but also to some degree in other ways (e.g. mass media). His developmental changes also have implications for the culture, again largely expressed via social participation in groups, but not entirely so.

The psychologist cannot ignore the extent to which the manifestations of adolescence are intimately related to the society and culture. In contrasting tribal society and modern urban society there are immense differences in the kinds of demands placed on adolescents; the range of choices open to them (4); the extent to which the adolescent has a clear place in society; and the extent to which the transition to adulthood is formally recognized (initiation rites, etc.). Within urban societies, young industrial and agricultural workers are likely to enter a fully adult role earlier, and more unambiguously, than their contemporaries who undertake long professional education and training.

MAJOR PSYCHOLOGICAL CHANGES OF ADOLESCENCE

Cognitive development

Central to the psychological changes occurring throughout development are the mechanisms of adaptation subsumed under the rubric of cognitive development. The major feature here is the progression from relatively automatic conditioned responses and trial and error learning of infancy and early childhood, to the acquisition of concepts and of a much more flexible and insightful understanding of the nature of the world in which he lives (47,48). This is greatly aided by the acquisition of speech and language. A very important step, typically occurring between 4 or 5 and 9 or 10 years, is the acquisition of what Piaget terms 'concrete operations'. This involves an understanding of reversibility of operations.

A younger child will be influenced by his perception of one aspect of the change, say height or width of the water. He cannot cope with the reciprocal relations between height and width (figure 4). The more cognitively advanced child can cope with this, and can recognize that the process is at least mentally reversible - that if the water in B is poured back into A it would reach the same level as before; that it is the same

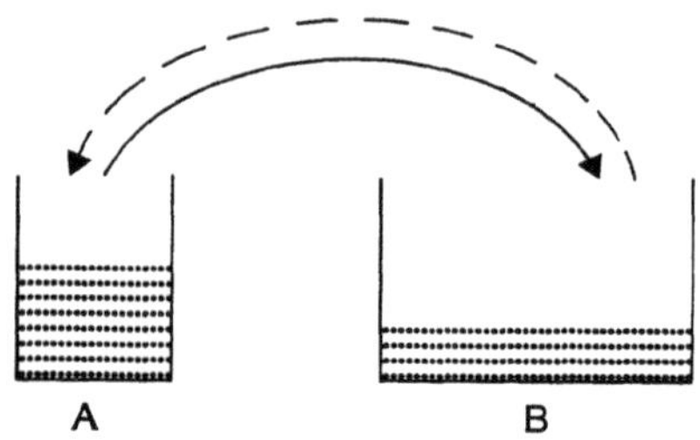

Figure 4. Liquid is poured from A to B. A younger child will think the amount of water is not the same, perhaps 'less, because the water does not come so high', or 'more, because it is wider'.

quantity of water. In other words, the child has come to realize that constancy can occur despite perceptual changes. Such a child is at the level of concrete operations, because he can only reason in this way with concrete material (glasses, water, cups, etc.).

A second major change in cognitive functioning normally occurs before or during puberty, that is the acquisition of 'formal operations' (Piaget). Now the youngster can deal with more abstract relations. Examples:

a) If A is bigger than B, and B is bigger than C, then A is bigger than C (This is the relation of transitivity).
b) If A + B = C, then C = A + B (Reversibility at the abstract level).

Hence, in the early teens the majority of children can begin to make sense of algebra, to understand principles and relationships, and reason about them. This has wide implications for secondary, as compared with primary, education. However, children who are still at the level of concrete operations will be unable to cope with more abstract teaching, and are likely to become disinterested in school, and even hostile to it, unless their needs are met.

Understanding of the world and society

This change in cognitive functioning also has implications as regards the child's understanding of the world, society, moral issues (49,50) etc. He can begin to see parallels and analogies. He searches for principles and rational explanations (51). He, therefore, in our kind of society, comes to question some of the assumptions of that society, to become aware of apparent logical contradictions. Examples would be:

a) The Bible says 'thou shalt not kill', why do priests bless soldiers?
b) You tell me that I should care about other people, so why is competition with them all right?
c) If socialists stand for equal rights, why don't the leaders take more notice of ordinary people?
d) Why is it bad to smoke cannabis, when you smoke tobacco?

It is easy to see how in an 'open society', where no one set of values is generally accepted, adolescents often find the adult world hard to understand and to accept. Thus, it is not surprising that some of them seek solutions in movements which appear to offer a solution, whether religious, social, or political. Others may opt out by becoming hippies, punks, or drug addicts. Increasing unemployment in western countries is likely to increase the questioning of assumptions, and the vigour of protests against them.

The position is in great contrast to that in stable, unchanging societies, where everyone 'knows' and accepts certain values as being beyond question, and in which such questioning would therefore be inconceivable.

Changes in social role and social skills

In coping with his changing social role, and the expectations of others, it is important for the adolescent to acquire both an understanding of other people and skills in interacting with them (2,37). Much of this will have been laid down in childhood, at first in interaction with the parents and siblings (52), and later with peers (53).

A major issue is that of the youngster accepting responsibility for his own actions, and of interacting with others as equals. Here there are often both internal and external conflicts, as indicated earlier. The school and various forms of social clubs, sports clubs, etc., can help a great deal in encouraging and fostering the ability to get on with others.

The self

Arising from conflicts between the child and adult roles, and from his cognitive development, it is not surprising that the youngster wants to know 'who am I', 'what am I', etc. (18,22). His own views of himself: good or bad, clever or stupid, kind or selfish, popular or unpopular, are affected by how other people (parents, teachers, peers) view him; by his own experience of doing things at school and elsewhere; and generally by his relationships with other people (23, chapter 14). Here, too, a positive attitude to himself can be helped by understanding teachers, youth leaders, etc., as well as by parents, if they see the importance of encouraging the development of his positive potentialities (2,54).

Intimately related to the youngster's view of himself is the extent to which he identifies with his own sex role. There is evidence that appropriate identification is favoured by a warm positive relationship with the parent of the same sex, and being valued as a young man or young woman by the parent of opposite sex (52,55). However, what constitutes appropriate identification is changing rapidly (2) and differs as between countries (56,57).

Occupational orientation

Insofar as adolescence is a preparation for adulthood, an

important task is to equip youngsters for a suitable occupation in the adult world. Such varied personal features as size and strength, sex, general and specific abilities, social skills, and personal values, all affect the outcome, which in turn is affected by parents, teachers, and the youngster's social background. Recent work by Moore indicates that adolescents' occupational aspirations are likely to undergo change, and become more realistic (58,59).

Again, identification with the like-sexed parent is an important factor, positively or negatively. When a youngster wants to adopt the same occupation as the parent, and has a close identification with him/her, then things are likely to be easier. A hostile relationship with the parent, and ambivalent identification, may lead a youngster to reject the parent's occupation (and values). There can also be problems when the child's ability level implies an occupation very different from that of the parent. Examples would be:

a) When a child of working class background does very well at school, pursuit of higher education and professional training may lead to conflicts with his/her identification with the parent, and with parental values.
b) Similarly, if a child of professional background is academically backward, and is therefore best suited for a manual occupation.

The researches of Douglas et al. (60) indicate clearly how family and social background commonly influence educational attainment among children of similar ability levels.

INFLUENCES OF PUBERTY ON PSYCHOLOGICAL DEVELOPMENT

Tanner (1,61) called attention to some association between precocity in physical development and level of I.Q., and between height in childhood and I.Q. This is of some theoretical interest, but the level of relationship is too small to have much practical relevance.

More direct effects of puberty on behaviour

Of much more obvious importance are the ways in which the physical and hormonal changes of puberty have both direct and indirect effects on behaviour.

Obviously, mature sexual behaviour depends on the maturity of the sex organs. The male cannot ejaculate until the genital apparatus is ready, nor is the female likely to be able to accommodate a normal penis before puberty. However, there is plenty of evidence of precursors of sexual behaviour in human children. Freud's insistence on what he termed 'infantile sexuality', and what might better be termed 'infantile eroticism', has been borne out by evidence of infants' pleasurable responses to stimulation of erogenous zones (62) and of apparent pleasure in detumescence (63). Western societies generally discourage overt sexual behaviour in childhood, but various forms of self-stimulation are a commonplace. Malinowski's (64) classic anthropological researches in the Melanesia of the 1920's do indicate that where such behaviour was not discouraged, not only would young children engage in sexual play, but boys of five years would penetrate little girls of a similar age. Mead's (6) findings were similar. Thus, it appears that humans are capable quite early of some of the aspects of mature sexual behaviour. This seems rather to contradict some of the work on lower mammals, among which it is known that their sexual behaviour is much more attributable to presence of hormones and to the immediate stimulation provided by a mature member of the opposite sex. In humans, sexual behaviour, as with other forms of behaviour, is greatly influenced by the culture and by fantasies, memories, and by such symbolic representations as literature, or music.

The systematic study of the development of sexual behaviour is very difficult in our kind of society, and we therefore have to rely to a large extent on the retrospective data collected by such workers as Kinsey (65,66) in the U.S.A., supplemented by the more recent studies on representative samples by Schofield (67,68) in Britain, and Zelnik and Kantner (69) in the U.S.A.

Although the accuracy of the data is open to some doubts, nevertheless certain tendencies appear: by 15 years the great majority of boys have had an orgasm (mostly from masturbation), and masturbation is the norm at this age; it seems that far fewer girls have had an orgasm by this age, and that they masturbate less frequently; more boys than girls have had sexual intercourse by 15 years; in both sexes the numbers having intercourse rise with age, so that by 21 years around 70% of both sexes have experienced it (67,68). Zelnik and Kantner's (69) figures for girls are similar, in that 55% of the unmarried had experienced intercourse by 19 years. It is of interest that these investigators and Schofield find that promiscuity is the exception rather than the norm (9). There is increasing recent evidence of change, particularly amongst girls. Several studies have now reported similar incidence of intercourse among boys and girls (70,71).

It is perhaps not surprising that both Kinsey et al. (65) and Schofield (67) reported more sexual activity in early maturing boys, and in Schofield's case in early maturing girls also. Kinsey provided evidence of a continuing greater frequency of later sexual behaviour in males who matured early. Conceivably such males differ from the rest in output of sex hormones.

Ausubel (19) commented on evidence of what he termed a psychosexual orientation in boys, compared with a more psycho-affectional orientation in girls. The latter were much more likely to have intercourse because they were in love, or to please their boy-friends. In the second edition (3) a less clear distinction is drawn between the sexes, and there seems generally to be a tendency towards greater similarity in attitudes and behaviour (72). Lerner and Spanier (9) conclude that boys are still much more likely to initiate sexual contacts than girls, but one suspects that here, too, change may be occurring. Certainly in considering evidence from primitive societies, Ausubel (19) referred to some in which females took sexual initiatives as commonly as males, which suggests a strong cultural component in this, as in other behaviour.

More indirect effects of puberty on behaviour

Here we are referring to the way in which his/her size, strength, and appearance as being physically mature, affects the adolescent's view of himself/herself, and the response of other people. In the case of boys, those who mature early are, of course, taller and stronger, and therefore are better at sport or at fighting. Not surprisingly they are more popular among peers, more likely to be seen as leaders, and more likely to be given responsibility by teachers. Late maturers tend to be less popular, and less sure of themselves (73,74).

Among girls, very early maturity can be a disadvantage, as precocious sexual development may not be welcomed by adults, and the girls may feel embarrassed about being the only one in the peer group who menstruates, or has breasts (75). The late maturing girl has the problems of wondering whether she is normal, as well as those of being less popular. Thus, girls somewhere near the norm are likely to have an easier time in this transition period.

CONCLUSION

This brief review has suggested that adolescence consists of a very complex set of changes. The society sets the scene, in determining how the changes of puberty will be responded to, and in determining the ways in which the transition from childhood to adulthood can be accomplished. How easily the transition occurs will then depend on the extent to which life in childhood has prepared the youngster to cope with it, on the way in which parents and the school system assist in the process, on the cognitive and social skills which the adolescent has acquired, and on the extent to which he is able to develop a self-concept which is appropriate to his own qualities in relation to his life situation.

REFERENCES

1. Tanner JM. 1962. Growth at adolescence (2nd edition). Oxford: Blackwell.
2. Conger JJ. 1977. Adolescence and youth: psychological development in a changing world. New York: Harper and Row.
3. Ausubel DP, Montemayor R, Svajian P. 1977. Theory and problems of adolescent development (2nd edition). New York: Grune and Stratton.
4. Wall WD. 1968. Adolescents in school and society. Slough: National Foundation for Educational Research.
5. Hall GS. 1904. Adolescence. New York: Appleton.
6. Mead M. 1928. Coming of age in Samoa. New York: Morrow.
7. Benedict R. 1938. Continuities and discontinuities in cultural conditioning. Psychiatry 1, 161-167.
8. Gallatin J. 1980. Theories of adolescence. In: Understanding adolescence (4th edition). Adams JF (ed). Boston: Allyn and Bacon.
9. Lerner RM, Spanier GB. 1980. Adolescent development: a life-span perspective. New York: McGraw-Hill.
10. Bandura A. 1969. Principles of behavior modification. New York: Holt, Rinehart and Winston.
11. Bandura A, Walters RH. 1959. Adolescent aggression. New York: Ronald Press.
12. Bandura A, Walters RH. 1963. Social learning and personality development. New York: Holt, Rinehart and Winston.
13. Freud S. 1953. Three essays on sexuality. In: Standard edition, vol. 7. London: Hogarth Press.
14. Fenichel O. 1945. The psychoanalytic theory of neurosis. New York: Norton.
15. Freud A. 1948. The ego and the mechanisms of defence. New York: International Universities Press.
16. Freud A. 1958. Adolescence. Psychoanalytic study of the child 13, 255-278.
17. Erikson E. 1950. Childhood and Society. New York: Norton.
18. Erikson E. 1968. Identity: youth and crisis. New York: Norton.
19. Ausubel DP. 1954. Theory and problems of adolescent development. New York: Grune and Stratton.
20. McCandless BR. 1970. Adolescents: behavior and development. Hinsdale, Illinois: Dryden Press.
21. Sullivan HS. 1953. The interpersonal theory of psychiatry. New York: Norton.
22. Lewin K. 1939. The field theory approach to adolescence. American Journal of Sociology 44, 868-897.
23. Dusek JB. 1977. Adolescent development and behavior. Chicago: Science Research Associates.
24. Spranger E. 1955. Psychologie des Jugendalters (24th edition). Heidelberg: Queller and Meyer.
25. Muuss R. 1975. Theories of adolescence (3rd edition). New York: Random House.

26. Offer D, Offer J. (1975). From teenage to young manhood. New York: Basic Books.
27. Waddington CH. 1961. The nature of life. London: Allen and Unwin.
28. Waddington CH. 1975. The evolution of an evolutionist (Chapter 26). Edinburgh: Edinburgh University Press.
29. Hindley CB. 1972. L'influence du développement physique sur le développement psychologique. In: Milieu et développement. Duyckaerts F. et al. Paris: Presses Universitaires de France.
30. Medawar PB, Medawar JS. 1977. The life science. London: Wildwood House.
31. Hebb DO. 1953. Heredity and environment in mammalian behavior. British Journal of Animal Behaviour 1, 43-47.
32. Hindley CB. 1980. Conceptual and methodological issues in the study of child development. London: Institute of Education.
33. Piaget J. 1971. Biology and knowledge. Edinburgh: Edinburgh University Press.
34. Krech D, Rosenzweig MR, Bennet EL. 1966. Environmental impoverishment, social isolation and changes in brain chemistry and anatomy. Physiology and Behavior 1, 99-104.
35. Levine S, Mullins RF. 1968. Hormones in infancy. In: Early experience and behavior. Newton G, Levine S (eds). Springfield, Illinois: Thomas.
36. Rosenzweig MR, Krech D, Bennet EL, Diamond MC. 1968. Modifying brain chemistry and anatomy by enrichment of impoverishment or experience. In: Early experience and behavior. Newton G, Levine S (eds). Springfield, Illinois: Thomas.
37. Havighurst RJ. 1953. Human development and education. London: Longmans.
38. Marshall WA, Tanner JM. 1969. Variations in the pattern of pubertal changes in girls. Archives of Diseases of Childhood 44, 291-303.
39. Marshall WA, Tanner JM. 1970. Variations in the pattern of pubertal changes in boys. Archives of Diseases of Childhood 45, 13-23.
40. Adler NT (ed). 1981. Neuroendocrinology of reproduction physiology and behavior. New York: Plenum Press.
41. Goldman BD. 1981. Puberty. In: Neuroendocrinology of reproduction physiology and behavior. Adler NT (ed). New York: Plenum Press.
42. Grumbach MM, Grave GD, Mayer FE. 1974. Control of the onset of puberty. New York: Wiley.
43. McCann S. 1981. CNS control of the pituitary: neurochemistry of hypothalamic releasing and inhibitory hormones. In: Neuroendocrinology of reproduction physiology and behavior. Adler NT (ed). New York: Plenum Press.
44. Harris GW. 1955. Neural control of the pituitary gland. London: Arnold.
45. Harris GW. 1961. The pituitary stalk and ovulation. In: Control of ovulation. Villee CA (ed). Oxford: Pergamon Press.

46. Vandenbergh JG. 1974. Social determinants of the onset of puberty in rodents. Journal of Sex Research 10, 181-193.
47. Boyle DC. 1969. A student's guide to Piaget. Oxford: Pergamon Press.
48. Piaget J, Inhelder B. 1969. The psychology of the child. London: Routledge and Kegan Paul.
49. Hoffman ML. 1980. Moral development in adolescence. In: Handbook of adolescent psychology. Adelson J (ed). New York: Wiley.
50. Kohlberg L. 1976. Moral stages and moralization. In: Moral development and behavior. Likona T (ed). New York: Holt, Rinehart and Winston.
51. Peel EA. 1973. The nature of adolescent judgement. London: Crosby, Lockwood, Staples.
52. Mussen PH, Conger JJ, Kagan J. 1979. Child development and personality (5th edition). New York: Harper and Row.
53. Coleman JC. 1974. Relationships in adolescence. London: Routledge and Kegan Paul.
54. Coopersmith S. 1967. The antecedents of self-esteem. San Francisco: Freeman.
55. Douvan E, Adelson J. 1966. The adolescent experience. New York: Wiley.
56. Bakan D. 1966. The duality of human existence. Chicago: Rand McNally.
57. Block JH. 1973. Conceptions of sex-roles: some cross-cultural and longitudinal perspectives. American Psychologist 28, 512-526.
58. Moore TW. 1977. School and the developing concepts of work, responsibility and freedom. Proceedings of the 4th Congress of the International Society for the Study of Behavioural Development.
59. Moore TW. 1981. Career patterns of young men and women. Psychological Reports, Aarhus, 6, no. 2.
60. Douglas JWB, Ross JM, Simpson HR. 1968. All our future. London: Davies.
61. Tanner JM. 1961. Education and physical growth. London: University of London Press.
62. Watson JB. 1919. Psychology from the standpoint of a behaviorist. Philadelphia: Lippincott.
63. Halverson HM. 1940. Genital and sphincter behavior of the male infant. Journal of Genetic Psychology 56, 95-136.
64. Malinowski B. 1927. Sex and repression in savage society. New York: Harcourt, Brace.
65. Kinsey AC, Pomeroy WB, Martin CE. 1948. Sexual behavior in the human male. Philadelphia: Saunders.
66. Kinsey AC, Pomeroy WB, Martin CE, Gebhard PH. 1953. Sexual behavior in the human female. Philadelphia: Saunders.
67. Schofield M. 1965. The sexual behaviour of young people. London: Longmans.
68. Schofield M. 1973. The sexual behaviour of young adults. London: Allen Lane.
69. Zelnik M, Kantner JF. 1977. Sexual and contraceptive experience of young unmarried women in the United States, 1976 and 1971. Family Planning Perspective 9, 55-71.

70. Miller PY, Simon W. 1974. Adolescent sexual behavior: context and change. Social problems 22, 58-76.
71. Vener AM, Stewart CS. 1974. Adolescent sexual behavior in Middle America revisited: 1970-1973. Journal of Marriage and Family 36, 728-735.
72. Miller PY, Simon W. 1980. The development of sexuality in adolescence. In: Handbook of adolescent psychology. Adelson J (ed). New York: Wiley.
73. Jones MC, Bayley N. 1950. Physical maturing among boys as related to behavior. Journal of Educational Psychology 41, 129-148.
74. Mussen PH, Jones MC. 1957. Self-conceptions and interpersonal attitudes of late- and early-maturing boys. Child Development 28, 249-256.
75. Jones MC, Mussen PH. 1958. Self-conceptions, motivations, and inter-personal attitudes of early and late-maturing girls. Child Development 29, 491-501.

4. THE PSYCHOBIOLOGY OF DEVELOPMENTAL BEHAVIOR DISORDERS

P.H. WOLFF

This report summarizes several studies on the neurological status of juvenile delinquents, and on the relation between learning disability and antisocial behavior at adolescence. Its primary objectives are to illustrate how biological and socio-economic factors interact to influence the course of deviant development, how such interactions can be investigated concretely, and why effective prevention and treatment ultimately depend on the physician's direct knowledge about such interactions.

Juvenile delinquency is a cultural concept whose boundaries are defined by local standards of socially acceptable behavior; and as such it has traditionally been the concern of judges and law enforcement agencies. Yet, many physicians are actively engaged in the diagnosis and treatment of antisocial behavior. They approach the phenomenon as a psychobiological disorder that transcends cultural boundaries; and they investigate its origins in terms of cytogenetic differences, perinatal stress and malnutrition, and brain damage. Biomedical studies have demonstrated that the sociocultural context alone is not sufficient to explain the origins of juvenile delinquency; but their ambiguous results leave it unclear by what mechanism biological variables cause antisocial behavior, or how identification of such variables leads to effective methods of prevention and treatment. Although an interactive formulation of the problem is evidently needed, the relevant biological and socio-environmental determinants of antisocial behavior are often so inextricably linked that their interactions have rarely been investigated.

Similar problems arise with respect to other behavior disorders of adolescence that are not in any obvious sense organic illnesses, but nevertheless come to the attention of the physician. School failure, for example, is in principle an educational concept whose boundaries are defined by historically changing societal demands for farmers, computer programmers, or cosmonauts. Yet, physicians are actively engaged in diagnosing and treating many children with school failure. They regard the phenomenon as a clinical entity that transcends historical circumstances; and they have expanded the concept of specific learning disability to include syndromes such as minimal brain dysfunction, hyperkinesis, and primary attentional disorders. Psychobiological investigations are useful in demonstrating that psychometric intelligence, motivation, and methods of instruction are not sufficient to explain the origins of school failure. Yet, they leave unanswered by what mechanisms neurological deficits cause school failure; or how findings from such studies can lead to more effective methods of treatment. As in the case of juvenile delinquency, the impact of specific biological deficits on learning disturbances in the classroom has rarely been examined.

More generally, a psychobiological approach to developmental disorders of adolescence raises questions concerning the process of human development whose answers may be self-evident in theory, yet are frequently overlooked in clinical practice. For example, what significance, if any, can be attributed to the observation that a discrete biological variable discriminates statistically between delinquent and non-delinquent adolescents? Does neurological impairment in boys who commit antisocial offenses indicate that they are inherently different from those who are not delinquent? And does it imply that detention is the only remedy until the appropriate drug therapy has been discovered? On the other hand, if we reject a simplistic biological explanation, does it follow that psychobiological factors are irrelevant to the origins of juvenile delinquency because the phenomenon is so closely tied to socio-economic conditions that it can only be contained by a restructuring of the society? While the interactive frame of reference is evidently preferable to both linear hypotheses, its utility depends on the ability to demonstrate how specific biological variables interact with particular socio-environmental variables; and how an understanding of such processes can be translated into feasible strategies of prevention or intervention - even if their scope is limited.

The point of departure for this report was a study on the incidence of choreatiform movements in children and adolescents with various behavior disturbances (1). The choreatiform syndrome is defined by small biphasic muscle jerks of brief duration that occur irregularly and arrhythmically in different muscle groups over the entire body. In children above the age of four, such movements are statistically associated with a history of perinatal distress, and may then be convenient behavioral markers for a subtle neurological injury in early childhood (2). The incidence of abnormal movements was examined in American and Japanese children of various ages, and found to be significantly more common in children with psychiatric disorders (47%), learning disabilities (28%), and a history of antisocial behavior (39%) than in normally functioning children of the same age and culture (11-12%). However, since the same minor neurological sign was also found in children without behavior disorders, choreatiform movements may be an incidental finding that has no demonstrable functional significance.

To examine the functional implications of choreatiform movements for skilled motor action, we carried out a second study by comparing the manual motor performance of 14 adolescent boys <u>with</u> unequivocal choreatiform movements and 14 delinquent boys <u>without</u> such movements. The motor task consisted of tapping as regularly as possible at the subject's preferred rate using fingers of both hands either in unison or in rhythmic alternation; and of tapping as fast as possible with the preferred hand. The maximum possible tapping speed did not discriminate between groups. However, all but one of the subjects without the neurological signs performed at a faster preferred rate and with greater stability of rhythm than did the boys with neurological signs. Apparently, choreatiform movements have a direct functional significance for serial order control in voluntary action.

The relevance of choreatiform movements for cognitive function was therefore examined in normal children by comparing academic achievement, psychometric intelligence, and classroom behavior of 10 to 12-year-old children from an affluent suburban community with the choreatiform sign, and an equal number of children matched for age, sex, and classroom placement who did not show the sign. All children were judged by their teachers to be good students: classroom behavior was scored on the basis of independent teacher ratings that had previously been entered into the child's cumulative school record. Even in this carefully selected sample, the presence of choreatiform movements was associated with subtle conduct disorders in the classroom, and specifically with teacher comments about the child's scholastic motivation, study habits, social maturity, and motor co-ordination, but the neurological sign was not correlated with either psychometric intelligence or academic achievement. In contrast, choreatiform movements are reported to be a common finding in children with identified learning disabilities. In other words, the same sign of minor neurological impairment which was associated only with subtle behavior disturbances in children who were preselected for good academic performance, may have a direct modifying effect on academic achievement in a less carefully selected sample.

Because the findings of the studies reported above were based on only a single neurological sign that reveals little about neuromotor function in general, the neurological and neuromotor status of adolescents with various behavior disorders was examined in greater detail by comparing the performance of adjudicated delinquents, boys in a residential school for learning disabilities, and normal boys matched for age, psychometric intelligence, and ethnic group, on the Lincoln-Ozeretsky Test of neuromotor maturity (3). The 36 items of gross and fine motor co-ordination were scored separately by independent observers. Results were summed across items as overall percentile scores; percentile scores were pooled across groups, rank ordered, and the rank order distributions computed (4). All but one boy in the control group scored above the 70th percentile for age on the motor test. In contrast, all delinquents, and all but one boy with learning disabilities, scored below the 5th percentile (chi^2=29.8; df 2; $p<.001$); and items involving rhythmic or sequential movements accounted for most of the variance in motor performance. Although the two clinical groups were indistinguishable on neuromotor criteria, they differed categorically with respect to socio-economic status even though the groups had been selected without regard for social class. Boys with learning disabilities came from middle class backgrounds, while boys detained as juvenile delinquents came exclusively from lower middle class circumstances. On the basis of these findings, we hypothesized that the same degree of neurological impairment may, in interaction with socio-economic status, induce either juvenile delinquency or learning disability; and that boys from lower class backgrounds who are identified as juvenile delinquents should manifest many of the functional deficits also found in non-delinquent boys with specific learning disabilities.

A more comprehensive investigation was therefore undertaken to examine the relation between juvenile delinquency and learning disability. Specifically, we compared the physical growth, neurological function, and neuropsychological performance: of juvenile delinquents from lower middle class backgrounds, non-delinquents from the same social class background, and non-delinquent boys from an upper middle class community, in order to isolate the effects associated with social class from those directly related to juvenile delinquency. The index group comprised 60 Caucasian boys from 14-16 years who were awaiting legal disposition or had been adjudicated as delinquents. Their court records were not consulted, but by self-report, the index group included approximately equal numbers of boys held for status offenses (truancy, vagrancy, stubborn child), boys detained for crimes against property, and those detained for crimes against persons. The two control groups and delinquents were matched for age, sex, and ethnic group. One control group comprised 48 boys from a school system in the same geographic area as the detention facility which had distinctly lower middle class demographic characteristics; the other group included 48 boys from an affluent community with homogeneous upper middle class demographic characteristics.

The full protocol included a paediatric physical examination, anthropometric measures of somatic growth and sexual maturation, an extended neurological examination, and an array of neuropsychological variables. The neurological component included the standard adult neurological examination, and items from the extended paediatric examination for minor neurological signs that are abnormal at any age, as well as for neuromaturational signs, such as associated movements and maneuvers of motor agility that are part of the normal child's motor repertory, which take on diagnostic significance only when they persist beyond a criterion age (5,6,7,8). The neurological examination included measures for hand preference, non-verbal intelligence, a protocol of language functions, measures of skilled motor performance, intersensory integration, attention, and spatial ability. The language protocol was subdivided into 'neurolinguistic' measures that are commonly affected in adult aphasic patients with localized cerebral lesions, and 'psycholinguistic' measures that probably reflect the social context of language acquisition more directly. The study has been reported in detail elsewhere (9), and only the relevant findings will be summarized here.

On neurological examination, juvenile delinquents showed more minor pathological signs and were slower and clumsier on timed motor maneuvers than either of the control groups. Lower middle class controls also showed more minor neurological signs than upper middle class controls. The associated movements were still sensitive to age effects, but delinquents were neither more nor less mature than other boys by criteria of neuromotor function, physical growth, or sexual development. The most striking result of the comparison was a pervasive language impairment in juvenile delinquents after group differences in non-verbal intelligence were controlled (10). Relative to both control groups, the delinquents showed significant deficits in word retrieval on the confrontation naming test (11); in syntactic comprehension on the Token Test (12); in rapid automatized naming on the Stroop Color Word Interference Test (13), and in the Peabody Reading Recognition and Picture Vocabulary Tests. Delinquents also made more errors of selective auditory attention (14) than controls, but there were no significant group differences on any non-verbal measure of neuropsychological function.

To test the relation between particular neurological variables and neuropsychological functions, we computed regression equations separately for each group, again controlling for age and non-verbal intelligence. In upper middle class boys, neither neurological nor neuromaturational signs correlated with psychological outcome measures. In delinquents, minor neurological signs correlated significantly with most of the language measures, but not with any non-verbal measures; and in lower middle class controls, neuromaturational signs correlated with several verbal and non-verbal measures, but neurological impairment was non-predictive. The magnitude of correlations was small, but the results support the conclusion that minor neurological impairment was specifically associated with language deficits in the delinquent, but not in other groups.

Self-reports about criminal behavior, although admittedly unreliable, were used to examine the relation between delinquency history and current neuropsychological status, because official court records themselves are often grossly biased. The self-reports were first classified by type, to include status offenses which are an historical anachronism that is not recognized in most penal codes, as well as crimes against property, and crimes against persons. By preliminary cross-tabulation, most boys currently detained for crimes against persons or property had been arrested for the first time before they were 11, whereas most status offenders were first arrested when they were 14 years or older. The incidence of minor neurological signs was also significantly greater in boys arrested for the first time before the age of 11, than in those who were first arrested at a relatively advanced age.

Thereafter, an arbitrary 'severity index' of antisocial behavior was computed by assigning different weights to status offenses (+1), crimes against property (+2), and crimes against persons (+3), and summing the weights over the various offenses reported by each boy. Neurological and neuropsychological variables were regressed on the severity index by a stepwise procedure. Language functions explained from 30-40% of the variation in severity of antisocial behavior, but neurological measures did not account for any of the residual variance after language performance was controlled. Therefore, if neurological impairment contributed to juvenile delinquency, it presumably did so by its influence on language performance.

DISCUSSION

In three separate studies, we found that adjudicated juvenile delinquency is significantly correlated with mild to moderate neurological impairment, across different neurological measures and in different comparison groups. The studies also indicated that among delinquents the neurological signs are directly related to impaired psychological function. Yet, neuromotor dysfunction was not a consistent finding in all delinquents; the same motor impairment was found in non-delinquent boys with specific learning disabilities; and among juvenile delinquents, the neurological impairment was not correlated with severity of antisocial behavior when language variables were controlled, whereas language deficits accounted for most of the variations in severity of antisocial behavior. Evidently, neurological impairment as such did not explain juvenile delinquency at adolescence.

Incidence studies by others have repeatedly demonstrated that the overwhelming majority of children officially designated as delinquents come from lower social class backgrounds (15,16). On the basis of epidemiological survey studies, one might therefore conclude that poverty is the necessary and sufficient cause of juvenile delinquency, whereas neurological impairment is a coincidental finding without any causal significance. Yet, the majority of poor children do not become delinquent (17,18); and middle class children, in fact, commit serious offenses against property or persons even though they may not appear in court records, institutions for juvenile offenders, or epidemiological census studies. Poverty undoubtedly plays an important role in the etiology of antisocial behavior and must be addressed on its own terms. Yet, socio-economic status <u>per se</u> does not explain the mechanism by which some but not other children of poor families become delinquent, or what is the cause of juvenile delinquency in middle class children.

One of our studies on children who were already diagnosed as having a behavior disorder indicated that the combined effects of neurological impairment and social class were important in determining the form of the disorder at adolescence - in other words, whether it was diagnosed as juvenile delinquency or specific learning disability. However, socio-economic status is a loosely defined descriptive term that subsumes a wide spectrum of concrete biological and experiential factors. Since each concrete parameter may interact with neurological impairment in a particular way to direct the course of deviant development, social class as such does not explain variations in behavioral outcome.

The third of our studies implied a more specific mechanism of linkage between social class, neurological deficits, juvenile delinquency, and specific learning disability. Severe language impairment discriminated efficiently between delinquents and non-delinquents either from the same or from upper middle class backgrounds. In the delinquency group, the language impairment was correlated with neurological deficits; and the severity of language impairment was directly related to severity of antisocial behavior. By the nature of their language deficits, delinquents were probably already at high risk for academic failure in the early elementary grades and before they were involved in antisocial behavior. Their performance profiles of severe language impairment and normal non-language functions were very similar to those of non-delinquent children with developmental dyslexia (19,20); and from a functional perspective, many of the delinquents were in effect children with specific learning disabilities. However, similarities in neuropsychological performance profiles do not explain by what process language-based academic failure in the early elementary grades resulted in antisocial behavior among boys in our group of delinquents, but does not have the same effect on other children from the same social class background who do not become delinquent. Presumably one or more additional variables intervened during the early school years that predisposed the affected children to antisocial behavior.

A brief psychiatric screening examination revealed that 70% of delinquents came from disorganized psychopathological families, and that many of them had not been living with either parent for several years, even when not in detention. In contrast, the majority of children in the control groups were living with both parents or with one divorced parent in a relatively stable home. Findings from the psychiatric screening examination are consistent with detailed sociopsychological studies which indicate that especially among the poor, family disorganization is a common correlate of antisocial behavior (16). Early detection and remedial intervention for academic difficulties in the primary grades can materially alter and sometimes correct the functional deficit of learning disability. Yet, the success of such intervention depends directly on active parental participation. Therefore, we hypothesized that children from lower social class backgrounds will be at high risk for chronic school failure, exclusion from school, and eventual exposure to an environment that is conducive to delinquent behavior, if they have a neurologically-based academic difficulty, and at the same time come from grossly disorganized families. On the other hand, children from the same socio-economic background with similar learning disabilities who have the support of their parents, or poor children from disorganized families who do not have specific learning disabilities, are less likely to be identified as juvenile delinquents at adolescence.

Finally, it should be emphasized that our hypothesis, as well as current views about juvenile delinquency in general, are based exclusively on studies of children from lower social class backgrounds. Yet, middle class adolescents commit crimes against persons and property, but tend to elude the juvenile justice system, so that they are rarely studied. A detailed psychobiological investigation of middle class offenders would nevertheless be of critical importance in sorting out the relative contributions of social class, neurological impairment, academic failure, and institutional neglect, as the necessary and sufficient causes of juvenile delinquency. It is quite possible, for example, that middle class offenders will not demonstrate the same severe language impairment; that the roots of delinquency differ qualitatively between middle and lower middle class offenders; and that different etiologies of antisocial behavior also require different programs of management and prevention.

The observations summarized above were limited to juvenile delinquents, and to only a small subset of all adolescents involved in antisocial behavior. Yet, juvenile delinquency also serves as a prototype for other developmental behavior disorders whose etiology cannot be located either in the biological or the sociocultural context alone, and whose medical management requires multifactorial remedies. In theory, the concept that behavioral development is always mutually determined by biology and experience is taken for granted. In clinical practice, the concept is commonly overlooked in favor of a single factor hypothesis, because it calls for time-consuming diagnostic explorations about the social context in which the disorder is manifested, and for a delicate balance between medical intervention and involvement of social support systems in the treatment programs which are usually not under the physician's control. The obligation to deal with such complex interactions nevertheless follows directly once we accept responsibility for the treatment of behavior disorders that were once the exclusive domain of judges and teachers.

REFERENCES

1. Wolff PH, Hurwitz I. 1966. The choreiform syndrome. Developmental Medicine and Child Neurology 8, 160-165.
2. Prechtl HFR, Stemmer CJ. 1962. The choreiform syndrome in children. Developmental Medicine and Child Neurology 4, 119-127.
3. Sloan W. 1954. The Lincoln-Ozeretsky motor development scale. Chicago: Stoelting.
4. Hurwitz I, Bibace RMA, Wolff PH, Rowbotham BM. 1972. Neuropsychological function of normal boys, delinquent boys, and boys with learning problems. Perceptual motor skills 35, 387-394.
5. Fog E, Fog M. 1963. Cerebral inhibition examined by associated movements. In: Minimal cerebral dysfunction. Bax M, MacKeith RC (eds). London: Heinemann.
6. Connolly K, Stratton P. 1968. Developmental changes in associated movements. Developmental Medicine and Child Neurology 10, 49-56.
7. Denckla MB. 1974. Development of coordination in normal children. Developmental Medicine and Child Neurology 16, 729-741.
8. Woods BI, Teuber HL. 1978. Mirror movements after childhood hemi-paresis. Neurology 28, 1152-1158.
9. Wolff PH, Waber D, Ferber R, Bauermeister M, Cohen C. 1982. The neuropsychological status of juvenile delinquent boys. Journal of Child Psychiatry and Psychology 23, 267-279.
10. IPAT (Institute of Personality and Ability Testing) Culture fair intelligence test. 1965. In: Mental measurement yearbook. Highland Park, New Jersey: Gryphon Press.
11. Goodglass H, Kaplan E. 1972. The assessment of aphasia and related disorders. London: Kimpton.
12. DeRenzi E, Vignolo LA. 1962. The token test: a sensitive test to detect receptor disturbances in aphasics. Brain 85, 665-678.
13. Comalli PE, Wapner S, Werner H. 1962. Interference effects of Stroop color-word test in childhood, adulthood and aging. Journal of Genetic Psychology 100, 47-53.
14. Doyle AB. 1973. Listening to distraction: a developmental study of selective attention. Journal of Experimental Child Psychology 15, 100-115.
15. Wolfgang ME, Figlio RM, Sellin T. 1972. Delinquency in a birth cohort. Chicago: University of Chicago Press.
16. Rutter M, Madge N. 1977. Cycles of disadvantage. London: Heinemann.
17. Werner EE, Bierman JM, French F, Simonoian K, Connor A, Smith R, Campbell M. 1968. Reproductive and environmental casualties: a report on the 10-year follow-up of the children of the Kauai pregnancy study. Pediatrics 42, 112-127.
18. Werner EE, Smith RS. 1977. Kauai's children come of age. Honolulu: The University Press of Hawaii.
19. Mattis S, French JH, Rapin I. 1975. Dyslexia in children

and young adults: three independent neurological syndromes. Developmental Medicine and Child Neurology 17, 150-163.
20. Denckla MB. 1979. Childhood learning disabilities. In: Clinical neuropsychology. Heilman KM, Valenstein E (eds). New York: Oxford University Press.

5. INFLUENCE OF EARLY EXPOSURE TO STEROID HORMONES ON BEHAVIORAL DEVELOPMENT

JUNE MACHOVER REINISCH

Prior to discussing the very limited research pertaining to the influence of early progestin and corticosteroid exposure on human development, it is necessary to review the much more substantial body of data regarding the effects of early administration of steroid hormones, especially androgens, on development. These data will be summarized in comparison to the normal sequence of events, with an emphasis on the ontogeny of sexual and sexually dimorphic non-reproduction-linked behavior. In addition, the wide-ranging effects of early steroid treatment upon the physiology and morphology of the brain and the body will be reviewed.

NORMAL DEVELOPMENT

There are several levels at which hormones present during early life influence development. Under normal conditions early exposure to androgen of testicular origin (testosterone being the most potent form) mediates the development of internal and external genital morphology, the structure and physiological functioning of the central nervous system, sexual behavior, and sexually dimorphic non-mating behavior. Finally, and most recently, there has been the suggestion that the presence of androgen during a critical period of development also affects the function of major organs such as the liver. Each of these systems appears to be influenced during a different stage, either prenatally or neonatally depending upon the species. Estrogens, exogenously introduced, have many effects paralleling those of the androgens; however, their presence or absence is probably not a critical factor during normal development, except as a product of testosterone in the brain.

The normal sequence of events influenced by pre- or neonatal steroid hormones is understood to commence with the production of testosterone by the early-differentiated testis. The introduction of this potent factor has its first effect on the internal genital primordia, which at this stage are virtually identical in male and female animals. The presence of testosterone and its metabolic products (in particular, dihydrotestosterone (1)) masculinizes the internal and then the external genital morphology (2,3). It has been found that the ovary remains undifferentiated until a much later time in development and has no known effect on its course during this period (3-10).

The basic pattern of differentiation in the absence of fetal gonads is feminine; the ovary plays no indispensable role in the development of female structures. Feminine differentiation appears to proceed in the absence of hormonal influence and at a later stage in development. On the contrary, the fetal testis is a very active endocrine organ that imposes masculinity against the basic feminine trend of the body (11). The presence of a masculinizing factor as essential for male development, and the absence of hormonal influence as essential for female development, is the core of the model for all dimorphic differentiation be it morphologic, physiologic, neural or behavioral. The majority of the evidence collected to date is based upon this premise and has been generated mainly from the rodent by either the removal of hormonal influence through castration of the male (or chemical interference with the present androgens), or introduction of exogenous hormones in the androgen-free animal (see review, 12).

Androgen influences on morphology and physiology

The dimorphic potential of the genital primordia is echoed later in development by a similar dimorphic potential in the central nervous system, also influenced by the presence of testosterone. In a series of studies beginning with Pfeiffer (13) in 1936 and continuing in the 1950's (14-16) it was determined that a part of the central nervous system was responsible for the cyclic or acyclic (tonic) pattern of gonadotropin release evident in female and male animals, respectively. This and subsequent research identified the hypothalamus as the structure responsible for the control of gonadotropin release from the pituitary (7,17-20). It appeared that the hypothalamus (at least in the rodent), like the genital primordia, was undifferentiated early in development (21). In the absence of androgen, the hypothalamus differentiates so that it maintains and regulates the secretion of gonadotropins from the anterior pituitary in a cyclic fashion, and thereby mediates the rhythmic cycle of follicle growth, ovulation, and corpora lutea formation, in the ovary, and controls the onset of menstruation or estrus (7). If androgen is present, the male pattern of tonic gonadotropin release develops (22), and if ovaries are present during maturity they remain in a constant state characterized by the presence of multiple follicles without any corpora lutea. Barraclough and Gorski (23), and Gorski and Barraclough (24), using brain-stimulation techniques, identified the preoptic-suprachiasmic area as the hypothalamic center responsible for the cyclic control of gonadotropin release, and suggested that it was here that androgen, during a critical period, had its effect, causing a loss of responsiveness to intrinsic or extrinsic stimulation. They placed the tonic control center in the ventromedial arcuate region. The above evidence on the hypothalamus suggested that just as the genitalia were undifferentiated during early development, the areas of the hypothalamus involved in the pattern of gonadotropin release (manifested dimorphically in adulthood) were also undifferentiated during early development. Further, it was the presence or absence of androgen during a set time in development which was responsible for instituting normal adult male and female hypothalamic regulation of the pituitary.

The manipulation of the early hormonal environment has further been shown to alter the physiology and physical appearance of treated animals. The presence of androgen during similar stages of early development altered weight, length, and oxygen consumption rate of female guinea pigs in the male direction (25); patterns of steroid metabolism in the liver of rats (26-29); and male rats, when castrated neonatally 'show female levels of plasma corticosterone following ether stress' which could be reversed by a single injection of androgen at the time of castration (30). The onset of puberty in females is delayed by exposure to androgens during early development, whether from an endogenous source (31, in mice) or experimental intervention (32, in the sheep; 33, in the rhesus). Finally, life span seems to be influenced by early exposure to androgens (34).

Androgen influences on central nervous system development

On the assumption that the brain underlies behavior, and that perhaps alteration of the structure and function of neural tissues could be identified in relation to the sex differences in patterns of gonadotropin release and behavior, identified as resulting from the presence or absence of androgen during early development, a number of careful studies on the central nervous system have been executed. The findings are in accord with expectation. Sex differences were observed between the brains of male and female rodents, and increasing evidence has been found that these differences can be manipulated by early hormone exposure.

Biochemical and physiological sex differences identified in the hypothalamus include: 1) oxidative metabolism (22,35-41); 2) protein content (42); 3) serotonin levels (43); 4) RNA metabolism (44); and 5) cholinesterase activity (45,46). Studies have also revealed sex differences in brain morphology which are mediated by early exposure to androgen. Sex differences have been identified with regard to: 1) nuclear volume in the anterior and ventromedial nucleus of the hypothalamus (47-50); 2) the dendritic field pattern of Golgi-stained neurons in the dorsomedial preoptic area, suggesting a sex difference in afferent input (51); 3) the neural connections from input of non-amygdaloid origin (52-54); and 4) the size of the medial preoptic nucleus (55). It has been suggested that hormonal influence on dimorphically expressed brain differences might not be limited only to the hypothalamus, and recent evidence supports this view. Hormone-dependent sex differences in nuclear volume (56,57) and oxygen consumption (41) have been demonstrated in the amygdala. Sex differences in the incorporation of (3H)-lysine (58), and cholinesterase activity (45) in the cerebellum, and DNA content (45) and oxygen consumption (41) in the cerebral cortex, have also been found. Finally, evidence of a hormone-dependent effect on the reaction to septal lesions, and subsequent emotionality, implicated limbic involvement in critical period neural differentiation by androgen (59). These findings lend credence to the hypothesis that hormone-dependent brain differences provide the foundation for more than just the sex differences in gonadotropin release and sexual behavior, but also provide the basis for sex differences in behavior which are not directly related to mating.

Androgen influences on sexual behavior

Sexual behavior has been shown to be affected by the presence or absence of androgen during early development. A large number of experiments demonstrate that depriving the male of testosterone, or the addition of androgen in the female, perinatally in short gestation animals, e.g., rats (5-7,10,44,60-64,251,252), hamsters (67), or prenatally in species with long gestations, e.g., guinea pigs (68), dogs (69), sheep (32), and monkeys (5,70), affects sexual behavior in a heterotypic direction. Deprived of testosterone, any animal, regardless of genetic constitution, will display augmented frequencies of female behaviors (e.g., lordosis) in adulthood, beyond the levels expected in the male (feminization). In many cases reduced male behavior is also a consequence (demasculinization). Conversely, male mating behaviors such as mounting, intromission, ejaculation and, at least in rats, ultrasonic postejaculatory vocalization, are greatly enhanced by the introduction of androgen during the critical period for the development of these behaviors (masculinization), with a parallel reduction in female sexual behavior (defeminization). Many of the above effects have been demonstrated in rats (6,49,61,65,71-75), mice (76), hamsters (77), guinea pigs (5,25,75,78), dogs (69) and rhesus monkeys (5,64,79).

Further, it has been shown that female rats, when treated with testosterone just after birth, 'exhibit a temporal patterning of male copulatory behavior identical to that of normal males' (80), even though the frequencies of some aspects of male behavior were lower than those seen in normal males. However, with pre- and neonatal, as well as adult testosterone treatment, 'females showed the characteristic behavior and temporal patterning of males both before and after ejaculation, postejaculatory vocalization and the normal postejaculatory intervals'. Sexual motivation as measured by 'the urge to seek contact with a vigorous male'(81), sexual attractiveness (10), and attraction to the male (in dogs, 82), are dimensions of sexual behavior which also seem to be affected. In general, the presence of testosterone early in development enhanced later male behavior, diminished the display of female behavior, sensitized the animal's response to androgen in adulthood, and inhibited responsiveness to estrogen and progesterone in later life.

Androgen influences on sexually dimorphic non-reproduction-linked behavior

There are many behaviors which are dimorphically expressed in male and female animals but are not directly related to mating. Investigation into the mechanisms underlying these differences suggested that many non-reproduction-linked dimorphic patterns were influenced by the presence or absence of androgen during critical stages in development, in a manner similar to that of the differentiation of genital morphology, many areas of the CNS, and sexual behavior. Among the behaviors which have been identified as related to early hormone exposure and are expressed dimorphically were: aggression (30,83-91); open-field behavior and emergence (10,67,92-94), running patterns (7); approach and allogrooming (95); avoidance acquisition (94,96); exploratory behavior (95); sleep patterns (97); saline intake (98); food intake and body weight (99-101); urination posture (69) and play and threat (64,75,78,83,102; see 12,103 for details).

ESTROGEN EXPOSURE: PHYSIOLOGIC AND PHARMACOLOGIC EFFECTS

A controversy exists today regarding the active agent responsible for either 'organizing' (7,25,75) or 'altering the responsiveness' (104,105) of the appropriate brain centers and the role of estrogen in this process. The traditional view has implicated fetal testosterone of testicular origin as the hormone which differentiated not only the internal and external genitalia but the brain as well. This view is held by a number of researchers including Goy (5), Harris (7), Jost (3,9,11), Phoenix et al. (25,64), and Young (106). However, it has been recognized for some time that exposure to estrogen (e.g., estradiol benzoate) neonatally, resulted in alterations (masculinization and/or defeminization) of hypothalamic function, sexual behavior, and sexually dimorphic non-mating behavior in female mice (107) and rats (7,19,21,108-115), which resembled those produced by androgen. Recently, a number of researchers have suggested that estrogen as a product of testosterone may be the active agent, at the level of the central nervous system, which actually mediates differentiation (116-119).

The argument supporting estrogen as the differentiating hormone is based upon the following evidence: 1) It has been shown that non-aromatizable androgens (those that cannot be converted into estrogen), like dihydrotestosterone, did not masculinize females (treated neonatally), or elicit masculine behavior from adult castrated male rats (120-122). 2) Estrogen plus dihydrotestosterone was capable of eliciting male behavior as fully as testosterone propionate in castrated males (121,123). 3) Androstenedione (an aromatizable androgen) has been demonstrated to be convertible to estrone by the brain (124,125). Further, Weisz and Gibbs (126) have shown that testosterone converted predominantly to estradiol, and androstenedione to estrone, in the hypothalamus of 7-day old rats. Conversion was greater in the infant rat than in the adult. 4) It has been demonstrated that the neonatal rat hypothalamus and limbic system possessed an enzyme system capable of converting androgen to estrogen (119). 5) Finally, rats treated neonatally with testosterone propionate and an estrogen antagonist (MER-25) did not exhibit the anovulatory syndrome typical of androgenized females (117).

One conclusion drawn from the above data was that 'the androgen effect on brain differentiation is via estrogenic metabolites formed at the site of action in the brain' (119). Following the investigation of three aromatizable androgens and five which were not, McDonald and Doughty (122) concluded: 'If exposure to oestrogen during the neonatal period is responsible for the suppression of female behavior, our results suggest that testosterone is the most effective means of supplying an oestrogenic precursor to the brain'.

If estrogen is the active agent at the level of the central nervous system, then it seems clear that it is not supplied in direct form from the periphery, since there is ample evidence to suggest that estrogen introduced neonatally in the rat reduces adult male sexual behavior (127,128). This finding has also been demonstrated in the pig with prenatal treatment (129). In addition, Feder et al. (130) found not only that treatment of experienced adult male castrates with estradiol benzoate and dihydrotestosterone propionate, elicited masculine mating behavior, but also that large numbers of treated animals displayed lordosis. Fifty, 86 and 92 per cent of the treated animals displayed lordosis, dependent upon the amount of estrogen administered, in contrast to only 9 per cent of castrated males treated with testosterone propionate and dihydrotestosterone propionate, and none of the intact untreated males of the strain. 'If male behavior could be activated by an appropriate estrogen treatment without concurrent activation of lordosis behavior this would constitute a stronger argument that the effects of estrogen on male behavior were of physiological significance' (130). It has also been reported that adult castrated male rats treated with testosterone plus anti-estrogen were capable of displaying masculine behavior (131) and that females treated with MER-25 (an anti-estrogen) displayed lower levels of lordosis, but simultaneously the anti-estrogen had a facilitatory effect upon mounting behavior (132). Finally, Feder and Wade (133) pointed out: Perinatal hormones decrease responsiveness to estrogen in the adult. It would seem uneconomical for perinatal males to produce substances that would decrease responsiveness to a required hormone in adulthood.

Although, as was noted above, critical period treatment of experimental female animals with estrogen resulted in masculinization of morphology, hypothalamic function, and behavior, a paradoxical effect has also been reported with estrogen - that is, demasculinization of the male. Greene et al. (134) showed that estrogen influenced morphological development of the male in the female direction, and of the female in the male direction, so that 'the result of the alterations in the development of the urogenital sinus is practically identical in the male and female offspring'. McLaclan and Newbold (135) showed that diethylstilbestrol (DES), a non-steroidal synthetic estrogen, when administered to pregnant rats from days 9-16 of gestation at 100 μg/kg/day, resulted in gross changes in the genital morphology of male mice. Diamond et al. (127) treated male rats with estrogen (estradiol dipropionate) perinatally and found that they 'demonstrated the strongest deficit in male sex behavior', when compared to controls and experimental groups treated with 9 other hormone preparations; 'showed female-like darting significantly more often than the control group'; and exhibited the shortest mean glans penis length of all groups. It can be concluded from the above evidence that whatever estrogen's role in normal physiological development and differentiation, when introduced exogenously during critical periods in early development, it had wide-ranging effects on the behavior, physiology, and morphology of the organism, in the direction of masculinizing (and/or defeminizing) females and feminizing (and/or demasculinizing) males.

NORMAL HUMAN PRENATAL HORMONE ENVIRONMENT

Although it seemed clear that testosterone produced by the fetal or neonatal testis was responsible for male differentiation of the genitalia, hypothalamus, and behavior in animals -including monkeys (33,136)- there was little evidence until recently to suggest that the human fetal testis was capable of synthesizing or forming testosterone at the appropriate time during development. It has now been demonstrated that the human fetal testis is able to form testosterone from C21 precursors as early as 8 to 10 weeks post-conception (1). The results of several similar studies (137,138) support these data and together demonstrate that this ability continues to rise to a maximum level at approximately 20 weeks, after which it declines until parturition. Studies of plasma testosterone have confirmed the *in vitro* evidence (139,140). When compared to males, female fetuses show no such concentrations or capability for testosterone formation. Abramovich (141) found the male levels to be 9 times those of females during weeks 12 to 18 of gestation, and remarked 'that the levels reached by some of the midpregnancy male fetuses were well within the normal adult male levels measured in this laboratory'. A study of concentrations of unconjugated testosterone in amniotic fluid from normal pregnancies of 9-40 weeks gestation also confirmed this sex difference (142). 'In two-thirds of samples from pregnancies with male fetuses, amniotic fluid testosterone exceeded the upper limit found in female samples with minimal overlap in the 12-18 week period of gestation'. Although the levels decreased toward the end of pregnancy, males continued to evidence higher testosterone levels in amniotic fluid samples. Robinson et al. (143) reported a similar sex difference in amniotic fluid between weeks 14-20 with no overlap of testosterone values. Androstenedione concentrations were also significantly higher in amniotic fluid samples from male fetuses. Doerner et al. (144) have demonstrated that peripheral blood samples from women only in their 7th to 10th week of bearing male fetuses, contained 'highly significantly increased plasma values of free testosterone', in contrast to those carrying female fetuses, although no difference was observed in bound testosterone. These findings have confirmed the presence of testosterone of testicular origin during the period of morphological differentiation of the genitalia in the human, and also well into the stage that has been suggested as the period of hypothalamic differentiation.

Of particular interest for the theory of gonadal hormone involvement in the development of individual differences in sex behavior and temperament, is the observation that there are individual differences in the level of testosterone among male fetuses at the same period of gestation. Resko (145) observed that some male rhesus fetuses had levels of testosterone in systemic circulation that were similar to those found in females, even though the majority of male levels were much higher. He concluded that 'our data support the hypothesis that during fetal development some male fetuses are exposed to more testosterone than others'. It is relevant to note that Warne et al. (142) demonstrated individual differences in human fetal male testosterone concentrations in amniotic fluid of as much as 20 ng/dl at the same period of gestation.

Summary

It now should be apparent that early exposure to gonadal steroids profoundly influences the substrata mediating male/female behavior, morphology, and physiology, throughout development. It should be noted that many of the effects produced experimentally in animals have been identified in human patients with chromosomal/genetic anomalies, resulting in abnormally high or low hormone levels during fetal development.

An example of a syndrome analogous to the animal experiments in which androgen is exogenously administered, is human females with adrenogenital syndrome. These females are born with masculinized genitalia resulting from high levels of adrenal androgen during gestation. A series of studies on these children throughout development has shown that the excess prenatal androgen not only affected morphology, but also influenced psychosexual and personality development (146-152). Conversely, patients with androgen insensitivity provide an example of human subjects whose endocrine status compares with the experimental animals deprived of hormone influences during early development. Androgen insensititvity, as its name implies, manifests itself as an inability of the cells to utilize the androgen produced by the testes of these patients, despite XY chromosomes. The result is the birth and development of chromosomal males whose external morphological appearance is female. They are usually reared unconditionally as females and are most likely to come to the attention of the medical community during adolescence, when menarche fails to occur. Studies carried out with these patients, at Johns Hopkins Hospital (153,154), demonstrated that they were very feminine in their attitudes, interests, behavior, and appearance.

This review has been presented in order to elucidate the far-reaching influences of early exposure to gonadal steroids on the entire course of development in mammals. Thus far, the natural course of events in which androgen plays the major role has been the focus of discussion. However, as will be considered in the subsequent section, our interest resides in the putative influence of certain steroids -progesterone, norethisterone (a synthetic progestin), and prednisone (a synthetic corticosteroid)- administered to pregnant women which, the limited evidence available suggests, have long-term developmental effects on the exposed offspring.

PROGESTINS

Evidence from two sources reveals that many of the synthetic oral progestins used for pregnancy maintenance have some androgenic potential. First, the chemical composition of some progestins is similar to methyltestosterone (an androgen) - possessing the 17-OH group in the beta position (155,156). Second, masculinization of the genitalia in a small percentage of female offspring of progestin treated pregnancies has been reported (156-164).

Progesterone and synthetic progestins in animals

Animal research supports the suggestion that treatment with some synthetic progestins during critical periods may have androgenic effects on females (11,134,165-174,250). Genital masculinization of the female rodent by treatment with synthetic progestin has been demonstrated for norlutin (174), norethisterone (170-172,175-178), norethisterone acetate (167,176,179), norethandrolone (171,176), medroxyprogesterone acetate (170-172,175-177,180,), and others. Most of these studies were carried out using prenatal treatment and, in the few cases in which behavior was evaluated, no effect was found (174).

Paradoxically, but parallel to the findings with estrogen, a number of studies have reported a feminizing or demasculinizing effect of progesterone and synthetic progestins on the male treated early in development. Genital changes towards the feminine have been demonstrated in rabbits (165) and rats with synthetic progestins (167) and progesterone (127,167). Neumann et al. (167) reported on a number of synthetic progestins which, when administered during days 15 or 17 of gestation to day 20 in the rat, produced both lengthening of anogenital distance (masculinization) in female offspring and shortening (feminization) in males. These compounds included: medroxyprogesterone acetate, norethisterone acetate, norethisterone ethenate, lynestrol, and norethinodrel. Hydroxyprogesterone acetate and progesterone feminized males without affecting females, and norethisterone, and DL Norgestrel masculinized females, with no data on the effects on males. Finally, Diamond et al. (127) reported the behavioral effects of progesterone administered to male rats on day 3 postnatal. Decreased frequency of intromissions and ejaculations was found. It is interesting to note that similar genital changes have been demonstrated in human males: Aarskog presented 5 cases of hypospadias in human males whose mothers had been treated with progestin during pregnancy (181,182).

Progesterone: putative protection against androgen

Testosterone is not the only hormone available during gestation and early postnatal life which shows a significant sex difference in concentration. Progesterone has been demonstrated to exist in significantly higher amounts in females as compared to males. Shapiro et al. (183) found ten times higher serum progesterone levels in 3-day-old female rat pups in comparison to males. Studies of progesterone levels during gestation in the rhesus monkey have revealed a similar sex difference (184,185). Resko (145) in an analysis of 33 male and 36 female rhesus fetuses from 59 to 163 days of gestation found a two-fold elevation of progesterone in the females. The significance of this difference was suggested by several investigations in which progesterone was shown to antagonize the masculinizing action of testosterone in neonatal rats (186,187). Resko (145) and Shapiro et al. (183) posited that progesterone, of placental or fetal adrenal origin, plays an active role in the development of the female brain by protecting the female fetus from circulating androgens. That is, the high levels of progesterone available to the female fetus may act as an anti-androgen during periods of development when the fetus is particularly sensitive to the masculinizing action of gonadal or adrenal androgens.

Progestins as teratogens

In the past few years, several large cohort and case-control studies of the consequences of maternal treatment with progestins and estrogens have revealed augmented frequencies of congenital defects in the exposed offspring. Heinonen et al. (188,189) reported on 1.042 progestin and/or estrogen-treated women, and 278 women who continued to take oral contraceptives during pregnancy, from a cohort of 50.282 births. As compared to unexposed children, in which the incidence of cardiovascular birth defects was 7.8 per 1000, children exposed to progestins and/or estrogens exhibited cardiovascular malformation at 18.2 per 1000, while the incidence of this defect in offspring exposed to oral contraceptives was 21.5 per 1000. The overall association of cardiovascular birth defects and prenatal exposure to progestins and estrogens was significant after statistically controlling for confounding factors.

Congenital heart defects are not the only malfunctions that have been associated with exposure to exogenous sex steroids.

VACTERL syndrome is a descriptive acronym for a pattern of multiple congenital anomalies (V=vertebral; A=anal; C=cardiac; T=tracheal; E=esophageal; R=renal; L=limb reduction) which has been identified as resulting from exposure to teratogens such as thalidomide. Nora et al. (180) interviewed all expectant mothers from July 1, 1973, to December 31, 1976, at Colorado General Hospital, and identified 143 consecutive patients with maternal exposure to hormones during the first trimester. For 118 of these, matched controls were obtained. Eleven of the 118 offspring exposed to progestins and estrogens during gestation had major malformations in comparison to 4 of 118 controls. Further, in case-control studies, the estimated relative risk of exhibiting components of VACTERL syndrome following maternal treatment with progestins and/or estrogen was 8.41, and the relative risk for congenital heart disease was 5.58 and 3.55. Dalton (190) did not mention any incidence of congenital malformation in her sample of progesterone-exposed children. In a review of prenatal and birth records of 600 treated pregnancies (191), one baby with congenital heart defects and one with limb malformations were observed. This represents a near normal incidence of congenital defects; however, only 71 (the subjects) of the 600 records were carefully reviewed. Finally, Meyer-Bahlburg et al. (192) mentioned one of 13 male subjects who had 'congenital heart defect associated with short stature and congenitally malformed feet'.

Ambani et al. (193) in their review noted, with regard to substantiation of an association between exposure to exogenous progestins and estrogens and congenital defects, that 'although there have been many reports during the last decade, it has been very difficult to document conclusively such a relationship', due particularly to questions about the choice of appropriate controls in the retrospective studies. However, they concluded, based upon the evidence to date, that it is reasonable to presume 'hormonal administration during ... pregnancy may be potentially teratogenic'.

PROGESTINS AND BEHAVIOR

There are several investigations conducted during the last 13 years which, when taken together, strongly suggest a relationship in humans between treatment with synthetic and naturally-occurring progestins and subsequent altered personality/temperament and elevated I.Q. or school achievement.

Androgenic progestins

Ehrhardt and Money (194) conducted the first behavioral study of offspring whose mothers were treated with hormones during pregnancy. Both personality and I.Q. were investigated in 10 girls exposed to synthetic androgenic progestins. Nine of the ten subjects were born with masculinized genitalia. The tenth was the treated sister of one of the masculinized patients. Analysis of the extensive interviews given to both the subjects and their mothers revealed an unusually high degree of 'tomboyism' in these treated subjects. Tomboyism was defined in terms of 'athletic energy; outdoor pursuits; and play with boys' toys, with minimal concern for feminine frills, doll play, baby care, and household chores'. Furthermore, the mean I.Q. of the groups, as measured by the Wechsler Intelligence Scale for Children, was 125, with a standard deviation of 11.8, as compared with the population norm of 100 (S.D. 15). Sixty per cent of the I.Q.'s were above 130, when only 2 per cent would be expected in this range from a random sampling of the normal population. These personality and I.Q. findings paralleled the results found in the studies of adrenogenital females (mentioned above). Although they tentatively concluded that their findings could be viewed as preliminary evidence of the effects of prenatal treatment with progestins on the central nervous sysem, due to small sample size and the concomitant possibility of sampling bias, Ehrhardt and Money cautioned against unrestrained interpretation of their data.

Progesterone

The second study was carried out in England. In 1968, Dalton (190) published data which lent added credence to the I.Q. findings of Ehrhardt and Money, and provided evidence on advancement of developmental milestones in children whose mothers were treated with progesterone for toxaemia of pregnancy. In the preliminary study, mothers evidencing pre-eclamptic toxaemia were 'allocated to the progesterone or control treatment group by random envelope method between the 16th and 28th week of pregnancy'. Examinations by physicians and questionnaires by mothers were completed at the child's first birthday. The sample included 29 progesterone-exposed offspring and 31 controls. Although there was no difference between the groups 'in the time of eruption of the first tooth, total number of teeth and talking ability', there was significant advancement by the progesterone-exposed children in the ability to stand unaided and walk unaided when compared to the controls.

Next, Dalton studied achievement ratings made by teachers of a different group of 29 children exposed to progesterone prenatally. The next child born in the labor ward of a normal pregnancy and delivery was used as a normal control, and the next child born of an untreated toxaemic mother served as toxaemic control. When the children were 9 to 10 years old, their: 'head teacher was asked to complete a form stating whether the named child was 'above', 'average', or 'below' standard in verbal reasoning, English, arithmetic, craftwork (practical ability) and physical education (co-ordination or movement and muscular control)'.

An analysis of the data collected on the three groups of children revealed that the prenatally progesterone-treated subjects received significantly more 'above average' grades than either of the control groups. The statistically significant better ratings received by the progesterone-treated subjects 'exceeded that of the controls by 10 per cent in all subjects, 14 per cent in academic subjects, 13 per cent verbal reasoning, 11 per cent English, 14 per cent arithmetic and 10 per cent craftwork'.

There is some question here of selection bias resulting from the differential selection of respondents for the comparison groups, as well as the concomitant problem present in using matching as a strategy for achieving pre-experimental equivalence of groups (195). Nevertheless, the effects were found to be both dose-dependent, and related to time of administration. Subjects receiving 8 g or more during gestation did significantly better than those receiving less than 8 g, and subjects treated prior to the 16th week received significantly higher ratings than those treated only after the 16th week post-conception.

Recently two reports of a follow-up study were presented which seem to confirm Dalton's (190) findings while providing additional information on personality development in progesterone-treated children (196,197). The new sample described in the Zussman et al. (197) report included some of the treated and control children from the 1968 investigation (now ten years older), and new progesterone-treated subjects from general medical practice. Controls were matched 'for sex, birthweight, SES [=socio-economic status], blood group, mother's age, and family size'. The authors began with a group of 65 progesterone-treated children and 96 children in the control group, ranging in age from 16 to 19 years. The majority of the families were identified as working-class. However, 'the final sample of subjects interviewed included only 30 progesterone children (12 females, 18 males) and 29 controls (12 females, 17 males)'. Additional sample characteristics included: mothers of the progesterone-treated subjects received a minimum of 500 milligrams progesterone during pregnancy 'for relief of symptoms of pre-eclamptic toxaemia'; duration of treatment spanned 1 to 34 weeks; and timing of initial treatment ranged from the 6th to the 39th week of pregnancy.

Results from the Differential Aptitude Test suggested that treated children showed a clear advantage in Numerical Ability. This advantage was significantly related to higher dosage and duration of treatment longer than 8 weeks. Responses to a retrospective interview on behavior from 5-10 years of age revealed the following significant results. Female subjects who received larger, longer, and earlier doses of progesterone, were 'less' likely to report having been a tomboy at this age. Progesterone females also reported having been more concerned with their appearance than controls, and early administration was associated with females having preferred long hair to short. Dosage, duration and early administration related negatively to reports of disciplinary action in school at this age for females, but positively for males. Higher doses and longer administration of progesterone were negatively associated with influence over peers at this age, particularly for females, while children with higher dosage reported playing in larger groups, particularly males. Activity, level of interests and play (athletic, outdoor, motile types of play) at age 5-10 was negatively associated with dosage and duration for both sexes.

Regarding current behavior, significant differences were found between progesterone-treated males and controls. These differences related to heterosexual activity and included: less daydreaming about girls; less dating; less time spent thinking about marriage and family life; decreased incidence of going steady; and an increased likelihood of receiving disciplinary action in school.

Zussman and associates drew two major conclusions from their results. First, 'that progesterone subjects are more studious and less socially interactive than controls'. This hypothesis, they maintained, was 'a more parsimonious and complete explanation for these data than a hypothesis of selective masculinization and feminization in different areas'. The second conclusion was that 'the evidence strongly supports the long-term influence of progesterone on the fetal brain, particularly with higher dosage, longer duration of administration, and early administration'.

Further discussion of the data and additional information was most recently provided by Dalton (196) in a sample of 34 progesterone-exposed subjects between ages 17-20 and 37 normal and 12 toxaemic controls. She reported that: Eleven of the 34 progesterone children obtained a university place compared with 2 normal controls and 1 toxaemic control, that is 32 per cent of the progesterone children compared with 6 per cent among all the control children ($p<.02$). The corresponding figures for 18-year-olds entering English universities in 1974 were 5.3 per cent for the inner London Borough of Haringey in which most of the children lived.

Most recently, Lynch et al. (198,248) reported on the evaluation of 15 progesterone-exposed offspring (2 males and 13 females), whose mothers were treated subsequent to the 16th week of pregnancy, and 11 unexposed controls (4 males and 7 females). Subjects were 14 to 17 years old at the time of testing. No differences were found on the WAIS, School Questionnaire, MMPI MF scale or the Embedded Figures Test. However, the WAIS was inappropriately administered to subjects under 16 (half the sample) and data were missing for some of the subjects on the School Questionnaire. A significant difference was obtained from the Eysenck Personality Inventory. The 13 progesterone-exposed females were significantly more introverted than the 7 female controls. An introvert was defined as 'being somebody who is quiet and retiring, introspective and fond of books rather than people, likes a well-ordered life and seldom behaves aggressively'. Although the sample size was quite small, and therefore, males could not be adequately analyzed; the treatment commenced late in pregnancy; and the appropriateness of the criteria for selection of controls is questionable; the finding of a significant personality effect in the exposed females is consistent with the evidence of studies cited above and in the following sections.

Medroxyprogesterone acetate

Ehrhardt et al. (199) and Meyer-Bahlburg et al. (192) recently reported preliminary findings from studies of 15 females and 13 males (mean age 11 years) exposed prenatally to medroxyprogesterone acetate (MPA), a synthetic progestin which is very similar in structure to naturally occurring progesterone. Exposed subjects were matched to controls on sex, race, birthdate (±6 months), and socio-economic status, and an attempt was made to match for vaginal bleeding during pregnancy. Treatment criteria included exposure for more than one week during the 2nd to 8th month from the last menstrual period (actual: 2-34 weeks). Total dosage of MPA treatment over the entire pregnancy ranged from a low of 140 mg to a high of 3.900 mg. No statistically significant differences were obtained in comparisons of MPA-exposed boys and controls. However, tendencies were reported: Exposed boys 1) 'were somewhat less intense in their energy expenditure'; and 2) 'showed less interest in marriage and having children' (192).

The study of girls exposed to MPA during gestation revealed the following results: 1) significantly 'more girls of the experimental group had a clear preference for attractive, stylish clothes, while most of the control group had either no preference, or clearly preferred jeans, pants and other unisex-type clothing'; and 2) 'a tendency for the MPA girls to be less frequently tomboys on a long-term basis than for control girls' (199). In addition, although not evident statistically, when questioned regarding activity, MPA-exposed females 'were more frequently described as falling into the categories of 'low' and 'average' in physical energy expenditure, rather than into 'above average' or 'intense' in outdoor active play.

The small number of statistically significant differences found between hormone-exposed subjects and controls may have been due to the low-dosage, short-duration treatment regimes of many of the pregnancies, particularly 3 of the 13 male concepti and 4 of the 15 females, in conjunction with small sample size. However, the descriptions of both male and female subjects exposed to medroxyprogesterone acetate in this study are consistent with the observations of Zussman et al. (197) regarding subjects exposed prenatally to high doses of progesterone.

These studies, while provocative, are by no means conclusive. However, all studies reviewed thus far which evaluated the effects of the exposure of human fetuses to exogenous hormones have obtained results indicating some significant effects on dimensions related to personality/temperament or gender identity.

Synthetic progestins: data from our laboratory

The following is a review of data collected by Reinisch (200) and Reinisch and Karow (191) which supports the contention that progestins may affect personality development in humans.

Six hundred records from two Los Angeles clinics and a private medical practice were reviewed. Thirty-four families were identified in which at least one pregnancy had been exposed to synthetic progestin and a minimum of one pregnancy had not been exposed to hormones. With these minimum requirements satisfied, all available offspring of each family were evaluated for inclusion in this study. In order to qualify for participation, the offspring of the treated and untreated pregnancies had to conform to the following criteria: 1) same parentage within families; 2) at least 5 years of age at time of study; and 3) complete doctor and hospital records on pregnancy and delivery. Thirty-six physicians and 50 hospitals across the U.S. furnished the pregnancy and delivery records for the unexposed siblings and additional information on the treated pregnancies. The criteria for qualification as a treated pregnancy were: 1) dosage: minimum of 450 mg progestin (range 525-9.890); 2) duration: at least 4 weeks (range 4-36); and 3) timing: treatment beginning in the first trimester of pregnancy. The 26 members of the progestin group were exposed to an average of 2.994 mg. The most generally administered hormone preparations were colprosterone, norlutin, delalutin, deluteval, provera, and provest. The mean age for exposed subjects was 12,46 years, while the mean age of unexposed siblings was 11.8 years at time of testing. Birth order was balanced between exposed and unexposed subjects.

Exposed and unexposed subjects were evaluated by testers who had no knowledge of the purposes of the study and the treatment category of the child. Each family was evaluated by one tester for consistency of measurement within families. Subjects were administered the age-appropriate Wechsler intelligence scale and Cattel Personality Questionnaire (201). These instruments were selected for their comparability of scores across age groups. In addition, a score was generated from the medical records to reflect the severity and number of prenatal and perinatal complications.

The results of an analysis of covariance revealed a significant effect of prenatal hormone exposure on subjects' responses to the personality measure. When progestin-exposed subjects were compared with their unexposed siblings within families, they were significantly more independent, individualistic, self-assured, and self-sufficient. An integration of these findings results in the characterization of the progestin-exposed subjects as 'inner' or 'self' directed.

The progestin group profile corresponds well to the findings of Ehrhardt and Money (194). The mothers of their progestin-exposed subjects reported high levels of self-assertive independence and self-reliance, and correspondingly low frequencies of dependency and demand for succorrance, when describing their offspring.

In contrast to the earlier report on 10 progestin-exposed genitally masculinized girls (194), there were no significant differences on any of the six scores generated from the Wechsler I.Q. tests. The full-scale I.Q. for the progestin-exposed subjects was 121.08 in comparison to 120.12 for their siblings. It appears that exposure to synthetic progestins has no effect on I.Q., neither augmenting nor diminishing scores, when exposed subjects are compared to the base line provided by the family. However, the scores of both exposed and unexposed subjects were 20 points higher than the norm, similar to the results obtained in the study of the 10 genitally masculinized subjects. The consistently elevated scores probably reflect the socio-economic status of these families who availed themselves of the expensive and time-consuming treatment to support at-risk pregnancy. (Seventy-six per cent of the families fell into the highest socio-economic categories, I and II, of the Hollingshead scale. No family was represented in the lowest category, V.) As would be expected, the best predictor of the later I.Q. scores of exposed subjects was the I.Q. of their siblings (r=.46).

There is, perhaps, an important difference in the samples used in these two studies which may be of significance. Nine of the 10 girls in the Johns Hopkins report (194) were masculinized morphologically by the prenatal hormone treatment. None of the subjects in the present study were so affected. It is possible that the exogenously introduced hormones given to the mothers in both these investigations would positively affect I.Q. only in children who were particularly sensitive to them. This fetal sensitivity might be signaled by the influence of the hormones on the genitalia. In other words, perhaps I.Q. is elevated only in children whose genitalia are also affected by the hormones, and not in exposed children who do not show genital masculinization. A second possibility is the differences between the progestins to which subjects were exposed in the two studies. The subjects in the 1967 (194) report were exposed to some of the most powerful and androgenic synthetic progestins -norlutin, ethisterone and ethinyltestosterone- while in the Reinisch study many of the progestins administered were not strongly androgenic in action. Perhaps only androgen-like progestins affect later I.Q.

development.

Finally, Cattell et al. (201) provide a configuration of six personality factors which research has identified as having a significant relationship to school achievement and success. The progestin group subjects exhibited high scores on three of these factors (individualistic, self-assured, and self-sufficient). Since no significant differences were found between exposed and unexposed siblings on the I.Q. test, the groups are in effect matched for I.Q. The prediction of higher school achievement in this sample of progestin-exposed subjects is consistent with the results from the British longitudinal study of prenatally progesterone-exposed subjects which demonstrated significantly higher school achievements from childhood through adolescence (190,196,197).

Most recently (202), an analysis of the scores of 17 pairs of females and 8 male pairs (each pair composed of one synthetic progestin-exposed subject and an unexposed same-sex sibling) generated from the Leifer-Roberts Response Hierarchy (203) revealed that prenatal exposure, especially to androgen-based progestins, was related to elevated physical-aggression responses (202). Exposure primarily to estrogenic hormones did not affect scores. These data tentatively suggest that prenatal exposure to certain steroid hormones may affect the later expression of aggression.

PREDNISONE

Effects on birth weight

Since their synthesis nearly three decades ago, corticosteroids have been administered for their anti-inflammatory, anti-allergic, and immuno-suppressant properties. They are prescribed routinely in the treatment of allergic and edematous states; collagen, ophthalmic, respiratory, neoplastic and gastro-intestinal diseases; and rheumatic, hematologic, and endocrine disorders (204,249). Serious threats to maternal well-being at times necessitate corticosteroid therapy during pregnancy (205-211). Moreover, adrenocortical hormones have been used expressly to induce ovulation and support pregnancy in women suffering from infertility (212-215). Thus both the deliberate and incidental treatment of pregnancy with corticosteroids have resulted in the exposure of large numbers of fetuses to augmented adrenal hormone levels.

The paucity of reports on the possible effects on the human fetus of these powerful substances is surprising. Those reports which do exist are based on small numbers of individuals and fall into one of two categories. In one type of study, subjects received relatively large amounts of corticosteroids for the alleviation of severe symptomatology unrelated to pregnancy (205-211). In the second type, the offspring were evaluated during clinical trials in which low doses of corticosteroids were administered over long periods for infertility and subsequent maintenance of pregnancy (155,212 214). In both types of experiments, little risk of exposure was noted for either mother or offspring, although somewhat higher frequencies of stillbirth and spontaneous abortion, as well as isolated instances of cleft palate, were occasionally reported (155,208-210).

These reports of negligible effects on the human fetus are in marked contrast to data derived from animals, in which exposure to corticosteroids during gestation apparently produces deleterious effects. Such effects as resorption, stillbirth, reduced weight and length, cleft palate, and decreased thymus weight, have been observed in chick embryos and mouse, rat and rabbit fetuses exposed to corticosteroids (205,216-223). However, the dosages administered in most of these investigations were proportionally higher than those used for therapeutic treatment in humans.

Since no study of human offspring exposed to low dosages of corticosteroids throughout gestation could be found, we initiated an evaluation of a large sample of offspring of women who were treated with corticosteroids for infertility and maintenance of pregnancy In any study of the offspring of women treated with drugs during pregnancy, the most serious confounding variable is the maternal disease or malfunction which necessitated the initiation of therapeutic intervention. This makes it difficult, if not impossible, to extricate the effects of the treatment from those of the maternal complaint. Therefore, in an effort to measure the possible effects on a healthy organism, we undertook a simultaneous study of laboratory animals treated with corticosteroids in dosages proportional to those given humans. Thus, if similar effects were obtained from the human and animal subjects, any observed consequences in the humans could be more confidently ascribed to the treatment.

The full-term offspring of all women who received prednisone during pregnancy (n=119), at a private southern California infertility clinic between 1955 and 1975, served as the experimental subjects. The women in this group received 10 mg of prednisone per day for infertility, and treatment was continued throughout pregnancy. Prednisone is a synthetic corticosteroid with a potency five times that of cortisone and has become the steroid of choice in clinical practice (204,249). The comparison group was composed of the offspring of 67 women from the same clinic population who did not receive prednisone or any other hormone therapy during this pregnancy, although hormonal support was administered during a previous or subsequent pregnancy. Thus, mothers of offspring from both the experimental and comparison groups were comparable in that they were subject to problems of infertility sometime during their reproductive lives.

A factorial analysis of variance revealed that offspring exposed prenatally to prednisone weighed significantly less than control offspring ($p < .0001$). The average weight of exposed neonates was 2920 g while the comparison group average was 3370 g. No difference was found between the birth weight of male and female neonates (224).

As mentioned above, we undertook an experiment with animals to add support to the assumption that the lowered birth weight of offspring exposed prenatally to prednisone was mediated by the hormonal intervention, and not by the clinical condition for which it was given. Pregnant female mice were treated with prednisone from days 13-18 of pregnancy in doses calculated to be proportional to that which the women received.

Separate analyses of variance were performed to compare weights at each of three fetal ages (days 14, 16, and 18) and at term. Significant effects were not observed on day 14. However, 16-day-old fetuses exposed to prednisone (either 100 or 400 μg) for only 4 days weighed significantly less than did controls ($p<.001$). Both the 18-day-old fetuses and the full-term pups exposed to either dose of the hormone also weighed less than did offspring of control mothers ($p<.001$). Further, no significant differences in weight between males and females were obtained. Multiple comparison procedures (Duncan's test) revealed that on days 16 and 18 and at term, animals exposed to 100 μg of prednisone weighed significantly less than did controls ($p<.05$). Finally, while not differing significantly on day 16, by day 18 and at term, the fetuses and pups exposed to 400 μg of prednisone weighed significantly less than those exposed to 100 μg ($p<.001$).

The results of these experiments indicate that the growth of offspring exposed to prednisone during gestation is significantly retarded and results in diminished full-term birth weight. Three explanations can be offered to describe the mechanisms by which prednisone affects fetal weight. First, since corticosteroids readily cross the placental barrier (225-229), the lowered weights observed may be the outcome of a direct effect upon the fetus. It is interesting in this regard that children treated with corticosteroids for the alleviation of asthmatic symptoms show evidence of severe growth retardation and suppression (230). Second, the effects may be mediated by placental abnormalities resulting from prednisone exposure. This possibility is supported by data demonstrating that adreno-corticosteroid-exposed placentae show decreased growth (231), and, in particular, glycogen depletion (218), in comparison to non-exposed placental tissue. Finally, it is also possible that a direct effect of exogenous corticosteroids on maternal physiology leads to a subsequent secondary influence on placental or fetal growth, or both. These explanations are not mutually exclusive since any combination of the three could theoretically be operating in concert.

'Light for dates'

In 1967 it was suggested that babies born at, or below, 2.500 g after a full-term pregnancy, be designated 'light for dates' (232), to distinguish them from low-birth-weight infants who were premature (233,234). Full-term babies born at these diminished weights have been identified as at-risk for the neonatal period as well as for later mental and physical development (232,235-240).

The incidence of 'light for dates' babies with no congenital anomalies has been estimated in various populations to lie between 1.04 and 2.0 per cent (233,235,241). Analysis of 'light for dates' births in our samples revealed the incidence to be 1.52 per cent (1/67) in the control group and 13.92 per cent (16/119) in the prednisone-exposed offspring, a statistically significant difference.

In response to the discovery of the significant number of 'light for dates' births in the prednisone-exposed group of human infants, a second analysis of variance was performed to determine if the significant difference between the experimental and control groups would persist with the extremely low-weight subjects removed. The analysis, with 'light for dates' subjects eliminated from both prednisone and control groups showed the hormone-exposed subjects were still significantly lighter (average weight 3045 g) than controls ($p < .0001$). This finding indicates that, although only 16 prednisone-exposed subjects were born at weights which fit the strictly defined criterion for 'light for dates', the majority of the experimental subjects were still born at weights lighter than would be expected. To illustrate the magnitude of intra-uterine growth retardation in the prednisone-exposed offspring, it was determined that with 'light for dates' subjects removed from both conditions, 60 per cent of the remaining hormone-exposed individuals fell below the 25th percentile of the unexposed group.

Prednisone and behavior

Based upon our identification of an effect on physical development of the fetus (224) and the body of work indicating diverse long-term behavioral and physiological sequellae of early exposure to certain steroid hormones in humans and animals (see above), developmental studies of mice exposed to prednisone prenatally were initiated to determine whether follow-up evaluation of similarly exposed humans might be profitable (242).

Pregnant female mice were treated with prednisone (100 μg) on days 13-18 of pregnancy. As previously reported (224), birth weight of the pups was reduced. Exposed pups caught up in weight to unexposed offspring by weaning on day 21. Tests of aggression were initiated on day 62 after ovariectomy and implantation of a silastic capsule containing testosterone on day 60. Analysis revealed that prenatal exposure to prednisone did not affect the latency to fight of male mice. In contrast, female mice exposed to the synthetic corticosteroid during fetal development fought more quickly in response to the testosterone treatment than did unexposed animals ($p < .001$). Thus, females exposed to prednisone in utero were more sensitive to the aggression-inducing property of testosterone as adults and, therefore, were masculinized in their response to adult testosterone treatment.

A similarly enhanced sensitivity to the male-behavior activating property of gonadal steroids has been demonstrated in mice exposed to testosterone prior to birth (243). Since prenatal exposure to androgens also disturbs the reproductive activities of female rodents (75), a second experiment was undertaken to ascertain whether administration of prednisone during pregnancy would affect the fertility, reproductive fitness, and/or maternal behavior, of the female offspring.

Pregnant females were given either 50 or 100 μg of prednisone on days 13-18 of pregnancy. Birth weight of offspring differed among the groups ($p < .001$), with pups born of mothers given the 100 μg dose of prednisone weighing significantly less than the young from either the 50 μg or control conditions. However, this deficit in weight was no longer present at weaning on day 21. On day 60 of life, the females were housed singly with sexually experienced R-S males for 10 days. The resulting litters from the prenatally prednisone-exposed and control females were weighed, culled to 3 female and 3 male pups, and returned to the dams. Each female was tested for maternal aggression on days 4-9 postpartum by placing an intact adult male into its cage for 5 minutes.

There was no difference in the proportion of animals from each group that mated successfully or in the number of animals that failed to lactate or killed their young. Furthermore, there was no difference in litter weights at birth or on day 9 postpartum. However, there was a marked difference in the proportion of animals that displayed postpartum aggression, an important component of maternal behavior. Significantly fewer mice born of mothers administered 100 μg prednisone during pregnancy attacked the intruder as compared to animals from 50 μg prednisone or control conditions (Chi Square, $p < .01$).

The results of these studies (242) demonstrated that prenatal exposure to prednisone significantly modified two characteristics of the female. First, female mice normally require an extended period of testosterone treatment during adulthood to induce male-like fighting behavior. Those exposed to prednisone prenatally responded much more rapidly to the aggression-activating property of testosterone than did controls. Second, lactating female mice generally attack conspecifics introduced into their home territory, presumably to protect the young. Female mice exposed to prednisone prior to birth were less likely to display maternal aggression, even though fertility, support of pregnancy, and lactation were indistinguishable from that seen in unexposed dams.

The effects described above may be either a specific consequence of prenatal exposure to prednisone or a product of reduced weight at birth. The latter possibility must be considered since the effects of prednisone were manifest only in females born of mothers administered 100 μg, a dosage which affects birth weight. This seems unlikely, however, because females born of mothers which were treated with ACTH during pregnancy, while lower in birth weight than control offspring, were unchanged in their sensitivity to testosterone as adults (244). Therefore, the observed effects, in all probability, were directly attributable to an influence of prednisone upon fetal development.

Other manipulations which elevate maternal and fetal corticosteroid levels (e.g. prepartum stress or ACTH administration) have feminized the sexual behavior of male progeny (66,245), and reduced their sensitivity to the activational property of androgen on fighting behavior (244). Female offspring were relatively unaffected by these manipulations. In contrast, prenatal exposure to prednisone enhanced the sensitivity of females to testosterone while leaving the males unchanged. Therefore, it seems probable that the alteration in sensitivity to testosterone which we have observed in females born of mothers treated with prednisone is not attributable to the corticosteroid-like activity of this compound.

Of particular interest is the similarity of prednisone to androgen in its effect on the response to testosterone in later life. Either steroid, when given prenatally, significantly enhances a female's subsequent sensitivity to the aggression-promoting property of testosterone. This strongly suggests that prednisone, in addition to its established corticosteroid-like activity, is in some manner androgenic. Supporting this suggestion is a recent report in which prednisone was observed to stimulate growth of the seminal vesicles, an androgen sensitive tissue (246).

Prenatal exposure to prednisone also reduced the probability that postpartum aggression would be exhibited. It has been shown that this behavior is initiated by stimulation of the teats by the young (247). Since lactation was unaffected in the experimental females, it would appear that a normal milk let-down reflex was present. Therefore, prenatal exposure to prednisone probably does not affect afferent input from the teats to the central nervous system. Thus, the absence of postpartum aggression in females exposed to prednisone prenatally may reflect developmental alterations in those areas of the brain which mediate the display of aggression by lactating animals.

In conclusion, prednisone, administered for the treatment of a wide variety of human ailments, has been shown to alter the normal course of development in mice when present during the prenatal period. Implied by this finding is a permanent effect of this synthetic corticoid on the central nervous system.

We believe the association of prenatal prednisone exposure with diminished birth weight -particularly the increased incidence of 'light for dates' babies- and the behavioral effects found in mice, strongly suggest that the evaluation of prednisone-exposed human offspring will reveal long-term influences on development.

CONCLUSIONS

Based upon the foregoing review of the long-term effects of early exposure to steroid hormones, it is apparent that exposure to these potent substances whether from an endogenous or exogenous source can influence many aspects of physiological, neurological, morphological and behavioral development. Many of these studies of human subjects have been, by necessity, impressionistic and lacking in the fundamentals of experimental design and methodology. Nevertheless, all the preliminary investigations strongly suggest that exposure to steroid hormones during gestation significantly affects human behavioral development.

ACKNOWLEDGMENTS

Original research reviewed was supported in part by grants from the National Institute of Mental Health (MH-30676), the National Institute of Education, the Ford Foundation, the Erickson Educational Foundation, Biomedical Research Support Grants (USPHS), and the Charles and Johanna Busch Memorial Fund (Rutgers University).

REFERENCES

1. Siiteri P, Wilson JD. 1974. Testosterone formation and metabolism during male sexual differentiation in the human embryo. Journal of Clinical Endocrinology and Metabolism 38, 113.
2. Burns RK. 1961. Role of hormones in the differentiation of sex. In: Sex and internal secretions (3rd edition). Young WC (ed). Baltimore: Williams and Wilkins, p. 76.
3. Jost A. 1972. A new look at the mechanisms controlling sex differentiation in mammals. Johns Hopkins Medical Journal 130, 38.
4. Clark HM. 1935. Sex differences in change in potency of anterior hypophysis following bilateral castration in newborn rats. Anatomical Record 61, 193.
5. Goy RW. 1970. Early hormonal influence on the development of sexual and sex-related behavior. In: Neurosciences: a study program. Quarlon GC, Melnechuk T, Schmitt FO (eds). New York: Rockefeller University Press.
6. Grady KL, Phoenix CH, Young WC. 1965. Role of the developing rat testis in differentiation of the neural tissues mediating mating behavior. Journal of Comparative and Physiological Psychology 59, 176.
7. Harris GW.1964. Sex hormones, brain development and brain function. Endocrinology 75, 627.
8. Jost A. 1953. Problems of fetal endocrinology: the gonadal and hypophyseal hormones. Recent Progress in Hormone Research 8, 379.
9. Jost A. 1973. Development and endocrinological aspects of sex differentiation. In: Birth defects. Motulsky AG, Lentz W (eds). Wenen: Proceedings of the Fourth International Conference.
10. Pfaff DW, Zigmond RW. 1971. Neonatal androgen effects of sexual and non-sexual behavior of adult rats tested under various hormone regimes. Neuroendocrinology 7, 129.
11. Jost A. 1973. Hormonal effects on fetal development: a survey. Clinical Pharmacology and Therapeutics 14, 714.
12. Reinisch JM. 1974. Fetal hormones, the brain, and human sex differences: a heuristic integrative review of the recent literature. Archives of Sexual Behavior 3, 51.
13. Pfeiffer CA. 1936. Sexual differences of the hypophysis and their determination by the gonads. American Journal of Anatomy 58, 195.
14. Harris GW, Jacobsohn D. 1952. Functional grafts of the anterior pituitary gland. Proceedings of the Royal Society of London B 139, 263.
15. Martinez C, Bittner JJ. 1956. Non-hypophyseal sex differences in estrous behavior of mice bearing pituitary grafts. Proceedings of the Society for Experimental Biology and Medicine 91, 506.
16. Segal SJ, Johnson DC. 1959. Absence of steroid hormones in the neural system: ovulation controlling mechanisms. Archives d'Anatomie 48 (suppl), 261.

17. Barraclough CA. 1961. Production of anovulatory, sterile rats by single injections of testosterone propionate. Endocrinology 68, 62.
18. Barraclough CA. 1966. Modification in the CNS regulation of reproduction after exposure of prepubertal rats to steroid hormones. Recent Progress in Hormone Research 22, 503.
19. Gorski RA, Wagner JE. 1965. Gonadal activity and sexual differentiation of the hypothalamus. Endocrinology 76, 226.
20. Schally AV, Kastin AJ. 1969. The present concept of the nature of hypothalamic hormones stimulating and inhibiting the release of pituitary hormones. Triangle 9, 19.
21. Gorski RA. 1973. Perinatal effects of sex steroids on brain development and function. In: Progress in Brain Research, volume 39. Zimmerman E, Gispen WH, Marks BH, de Wied D (eds). Amsterdam: Elsevier.
22. Moguilevsky JA, Libertun C, Schiaffini O, Scacchi P. 1969. Metabolic evidence of the sexual differentiation of hypothalamus. Neuroendocrinology 4, 264.
23. Barraclough CA, Gorski RA. 1961. Evidence that the hypothalamus is responsible for androgen-induced sterility in the female rat. Endocrinology 68, 68.
24. Gorski R, Barraclough A. 1963. Effects of low dosages of androgen on the differentiation of hypothalamic regulatory control of ovulation in the rat. Endocrinology 73, 210.
25. Phoenix CH, Goy RW, Gerall AA, Young WC. 1959. Organizing action of prenatally administered testosterone propionate on the tissues mediating mating behavior in the female guinea pig. Endocrinology 65, 369.
26. Denef C. 1973. Differentiation of steroid metabolism in the rat and mechanisms of neonatal androgen action. Enzyme 15, 254.
27. Denef C, DeMoor P. 1970. Sexual differentiation in the liver metabolism of steroid hormones organized by testosterone at birth. Annales d'Endocrinologie (Paris) 31, 785.
28. Gustafsson JA, Eneroth P, Pousette A, Skett P, Sonnenschein C, Stenberg A, Ahlèn A. 1977. Programming and differentiation of rat liver enzymes. Journal of Steroid Biochemistry 8, 429.
29. Gustafsson JA, Stenberg A. 1976. Specificity of neonatal androgen-induced imprinting of hepatic steroid metabolism in rats. Science 191, 203.
30. Levine S. 1970. The influence of hormones in infancy on central nervous system organization. In: Les hormones et le comportement: problèmes actuels d'endocrinologie et de nutrition (séries 14). Klotz HP (ed). Paris: Expansion Scientifique.
31. McDermott NJ, Gandelman R, Reinisch JM. 1978. Contiguity to male fetuses influences ano-genital distance and time of vaginal opening in mice. Physiology and Behavior 20, 661.
32. Clarke IJ. 1977. The sexual behavior of prenatally androgenized ewes observed in the field. Journal of Reproduction and Fertility 49, 311.

33. Resko JA. 1974. The relationship between fetal hormones and the differentiation of the central nervous system in primates. In: Reproductive behavior. Montagna W, Sadler WA (eds). New York: Plenum, p. 211.
34. Doerner G, Hinz G. 1975. Androgen dependent brain differentiation and life span. Endokrinologie 65, 378.
35. Moguilevsky JA. 1966. Effect of testosterone in vitro on the oxygen uptake of different hypothalamic areas. Acta Physiologica Latino-Americana 16, 353.
36. Moguilevsky JA, Libertun C, Schiaffini O, Szwarcfarb B. 1968. Sexual differences in hypothalamic metabolism. Neuroendocrinology 3, 193.
37. Moguilevsky JA, Malinow RW. 1964. Endogenous oxygen uptake of the hypothalamus in female rats. American Journal of Physiology 206, 855.
38. Moguilevsky JA, Rubinstein L. 1967. Glycolytic and oxidative metabolism of hypothalamic areas in prepubertal and androgenized rats. Neuroendocrinology 2, 213.
39. Moguilevsky JA, Schiaffine O, Foglia V. 1966. Effect of castration on the oxygen uptake of different parts of the hypothalamus. Life Sciences 5, 447.
40. Moguilevsky JA, Timiras PS, GEEL S. 1964. Oxygen consumption and carbon dioxide production in the hypothalamus and cerebral cortex: influence of sexual maturation in male rats. Acta Physiologica Latino-Americana 14, 207.
41. Peng M-T, Peng Y-I, Chen F-N. 1977. Age-dependent changes in the oxygen consumption of the cerebral cortex, hypothalamus, hippocampus, and amygdaloid in rats. Journal of Gerontology 5, 517.
42. Scacchi P, Moguilevsky JA, Libertun C, Christot J. 1970. Sexual differences in protein content of the hypothalamus in rats. Proceedings of the Society for Experimental Biology and Medicine 133, 845.
43. Ladosky W, Gaziri LCJ. 1970. Brain serotonin and sexual differentiation of the nervous system. Neuroendocrinology 6, 168.
44. Clayton RB, Kogura J, Kraemer HC. 1970. Sexual differentiation of the brain: effects of testosterone on brain RNA metabolism in new born female rats. Nature 226, 810.
45. Clark CVH, Vernadakis A. 1971. Sex differences in brain deoxyribonucleic acid and cholinesterase activity in rats. American Journal of Physiology 220, 1775.
46. Libertun C, Timiras PS, Kragt CL. 1973. Sexual differences in the hypothalamic cholinergic system before and after puberty: inductory effect of testosterone. Neuroendocrinology 12, 73.
47. Doerner G, Staudt J. 1968. Structural changes in the preoptic anterior hypothalamic area of the male rat following neonatal castration and androgen substitution. Neuroendocrinology 3, 136.

48. Doerner G, Staudt J. 1969. Perinatal structural sex differentiation of the hypothalamus in rats. Neuroendocrinology 5, 103.
49. Doerner G, Staudt J. 1969. Structural changes in the hypothalamic ventromedial nucleus of the male rat following neonatal castration and androgen treatment. Neuroendocrinology 4, 278.
50. Staudt VJ, Doerner G, Doll R, Blose J. 1973. Geschlechtsspezifische morphologische Unterschiede im Nucleus arcuatus und praemamillaris ventralis der Ratte. Endokrinologie 62, 234.
51. Greenough WT, Carter CS, Steerman C, DeVoogd J. 1977. Sexual dimorphism in the dendritic field pattern of Golgi-stained neurons in the dorsomedial preoptic area. Brain Research 126, 63.
52. Raisman G. 1974. Evidence for a sex difference in the neuropil of the rat preoptive area and its importance for the study of sexually dimorphic function. Aggression 52, 42.
53. Raisman G, Field PM. 1971. Sexual dimorphism in the preoptic area of the rat. Science 173, 731.
54. Raisman G, Field PM. 1973. Sexual dimorphism in the neuropil of the preoptic area of the rat and its dependence on neonatal androgen. Brain Research 54, 1.
55. Gorski RA, Harlan RE, Christensen LW. 1977. Perinatal hormonal exposure and the development of neuroendocrine regulatory processes. Journal of Toxicology and Environmental Health 3, 97.
56. Butenik GA, Brown GM. 1973. Morphologic sex differences in primate brain areas involved in regulation of reproductive activity. Specialia 15, 619.
57. Staudt J, Doerner G. 1978. Nuclear volume in the central and medial amygdala. Endokrinologie 67, 296.
58. Litteria M, Thorner MW. 1974. Inhibition of the incorporation of (3H) lysine in the Purkinje cells of the adult female rat after neonatal androgenization. Brain Research 69, 170.
59. Phillips AG, Deol G. 1973. Neonatal gonadal hormone manipulation and emotionality following septal lesions in weaning rats. Brain research 60, 55.
60. Harris GW, Levine S. 1965. Sexual differentiation of the brain and its experimental control. Journal of Physiology 181, 379.
61. Levine S. 1966. Sex differences in the brain. Scientific American 214, 84.
62. Nadler RD. 1969. Differentiation of the capacity for male sexual behavior in the rat. Hormones and Behavior 1, 53.
63. Neumann F, Elger W, Steinbeck H. 1970. Antiandrogens and reproductive development. Philosophical Transactions of the Royal Society of London B 259, 179.
64. Phoenix CH, Goy RW, Resko JA. 1968. Psychosexual differentiation as a function of androgenic stimulation. In: Perspectives in reproduction and sexual behavior. Diamond M (ed). Bloomington: Indiana University Press.

65. Ward IL. 1969. Differential effect of pre- and postnatal androgen on the sexual behavior of intact and spayed female rats. Hormones and Behavior 1, 25.
66. Ward IL. 1972. Prenatal stress feminizes and demasculinizes the behavior of males. Science 175, 82.
67. Swanson HH. 1967. Alternation of sex-typical behaviour of hamsters in open field and emergence tests by neo-natal administration of androgen or oestrogen. Animal Behaviour 15, 209.
68. Etzel V, Schenck B, Neumann F. 1974. Influence of cyproterone acetate during pregnancy on the sexual behavior of male guinea-pigs Journal of Reproduction and Fertility 37, 315.
69. Beach FA. 1975. Hormonal modification of sexually dimorphic behavior. Psychoneuroendocrinology 1, 3.
70. Goy RW, Goldfoot DA. 1974. Experimental and hormonal factors influencing development of sexual behavior in the male rhesus monkey. In: The neurosciences: third study program. Schmitt FO, Worden FG (eds). Cambridge, Mass : MIT Press.
71. Barraclough CA, Gorski RA. 1962. Studies on mating behaviour in the androgen-sterilized rat in relation to hypothalamic regulation of sexual behaviour. Journal of Endocrinology 25, 175.
72. Soedersten P. 1973. Increased mounting behavior in the female rat following a single neonatal injection of testosterone propionate. Hormones and Behavior 4, 1.
73. Ward IL, Renz FJ. 1972. Consequences of perinatal hormone manipulation on the adult sexual behavior of female rats. Journal of Comparative and Physiological Psychology 78, 349.
74. Whalen RE, Rezek DL. 1974. Inhibition of lordosis in female rats by subcutaneous implants of testosterone, androstenedione, or dihydrotestosterone in infancy. Hormones and Behavior 5, 125.
75. Young WC, Goy RW, Phoenix CH. 1964. Hormones and sexual behavior. Science 143, 212.
76. Manning A, McGill TE. 1974. Neonatal androgen and sexual behavior in female mice. Hormones and Behavior 5, 19.
77. Swanson HH, Crossley DA. 1971. Sexual behavior in the golden hamster and its modification by neonatal administration of testosterone propionate. In: Hormones in behavior. Hamburgh M, Barrington EJ (eds). New York: Appleton-Century-Crofts, p. 667.
78. Goy RW. 1970. Experimental control of psychosexuality. Philosophical Transactions of the Royal Society of London B 259, 149.
79. Phoenix CH. 1974. Prenatal testosterone in the non-human primate and its consequences for behavior. In: Sex differences in behavior. Friedman RC, Richart RM, Vande Wiele RL (eds). New York: Wiley.
80. Sachs BD, Pollak EI, Schoelch Krieger M Barfield RJ. 1973. Sexual behavior: normal male patterning in androgenized female rats. Science 181, 770.

81. Meyerson BJ, Lindstrom L. 1973. Sexual motivation in the neonatally androgen-treated female rat. Hormones and Behavior 2, 34.
82. Beach FA, Johnson AI, Anisko JJ, Dunbar IF. 1977. Hormonal control of sexual attraction in pseudohermaphroditic female dogs. Journal of Comparative and Physiological Psychology 91, 711.
83. Beanninger R. 1974. Effects of day 1 castration on aggressive behaviors of rats. Bulletin of the Psychonomic Society 3, 189.
84. Bronson FH, Desjardins C. 1970. Neonatal androgen administration and adult aggressiveness in female mice. General and Comparative Endocrinology 15, 320.
85. Edwards DA. 1968. Mice: fighting by neonatally androgenized females. Science 161, 1027.
86. Edwards DA. 1969. Early androgen stimulation and aggressive behavior in male and female mice. Physiology and Behavior 4, 333.
87. Edwards DA. 1970. Post-neonatal androgenization and adult aggressive behavior in female mice. Physiology and Behavior 5, 465.
88. Gandelman R, vom Saal FS, Reinisch JM. 1977. Contiguity to male foetuses affects morphology and behavior of female mice. Nature 266, 722.
89. Vale JR, Ray D, Vale C. 1972. The interaction of genotype and exogenous neonatal androgen: agonistic behavior in female mice. Behavioral Biology 7, 321.
90. Vale JR, Ray D, Vale CA. 1973. The interaction of genotype and exogenous neonatal androgen and estrogen: sex behavior in female mice. Developmental Psychobiology 6, 319.
91. vom Saal FS, Gandelman R, Svare B. 1976. Time of neonatal androgen exposure influences length of testosterone treatment required to induce aggression in adult male and female mice. Behavioral Biology 17, 392.
92. Blizard D, Denef C. 1973. Neonatal androgen effects on open field activity and sexual behavior in the female rat: the modifying influence of ovarian secretions during development. Physiology and Behavior 11, 65.
93. Denti A, Negroni JA. 1975. Activity and learning in neonatally hormone treated rats. Acta Physiologica Latino-Americana 25, 99.
94. Scouten CW, Grotelueschen LK, Beatty WW. 1975. Androgenic properties and the organization of sex differences in active avoidànce behavior in the rat. Journal of Comparative and Physiological Psychology 88, 264.
95. Quadagno DM, Shryne J, Anderson C, Gorski RA. 1972. Influence of gonadal hormones on social, sexual, emergence, and open field behaviour in the rat. Animal Behaviour 20, 732.
96. Beatty WW, Beatty PA. 1970. Effects of neonatal testosterone on the acquisition of an active avoidance response in genotypically female rats. Psychonomic Science 19, 315.

97. Branchey L, Branchey M, Nadler RD. 1973. Effects of sex hormones on sleep patterns of male rats gonadectomized in adulthood and in the neonatal period. Physiology and Behavior 11, 609.
98. Krecek J. 1973. Sex differences in salt taste: the effect of testosterone. Physiology and Behavior 10, 683.
99. Nance DM, Gorski RA. 1975. Neurohormonal determinants of sex differences in the hypothalamic regulation of feeding behavior and body weight in the rat. Pharmacology, Biochemistry and Behavior 3 (suppl. 1), 155.
100. Tarttelin MF, Shryne JE, Gorski RA. 1975. Patterns of body weight change in rats following neonatal hormone manipulation: a 'critical period' for androgen-induced growth increases. Acta Endocrinologica 79, 177.
101. Wade GN. 1972. Gonadal hormones and behavioral regulation of body weight. Physiology and Behavior 8, 523.
102. Goy RW. 1968. Organizing effects of androgen on the behavior of rhesus monkeys. In: Endocrinology and human behavior. Michael RP (ed). London: Oxford University Press.
103. Reinisch JM. 1976. Effect of prenatal hormone exposure on physical and psychological development in humans and animals: with a note on the state of the field. In: Hormones and psychopathology. Sacher E (ed). New York: Raven Press, p. 69.
104. Beach FA. 1945. Bisexual mating behavior in the male rat: effects of castration and hormone administration. Physiological Zoology 18, 390.
105. Beach FA. 1971. Hormonal factors controlling the differentiation, development, and display of copulatory behavior in the ramstergig and related species. In: Biopsychology of development Tobach E, Aronson LR, Shaw E (eds). New York: Academic Press.
106. Young WC. 1967. Prenatal gonadal hormones and behavior in the adult. Proceedings of the American Psychopathological Association 55, 173.
107. Edwards DA, Herndon J. 1970. Neonatal estrogen stimulation and aggressive behavior in female mice. Physiology and Behavior 5, 993.
108. Doerner G. 1970. The influence of sex hormones during the hypothalamic differentiation and maturation phases on gonadal function and sexual behavior during the hypothalamic functional phase. Endokrinologie 56, 280.
109. Doerner G. 1976. Hormones and brain differentiation. Amsterdam: Elsevier.
110. Doerner G, Docke F, Hinz G. 1971. Paradoxical effects of estrogen on brain differentiation. Neuroendocrinology 7, 146.
111. Doughty C, Booth JE, McDonald PG, Parrott RF. 1975. Effects of oestradiol-17beta, oestradiol benzoate and the synthetic oestrogen RU 2858 on sexual differentiation in the neonatal female rat. Journal of Endocrinology 67, 419.

112. Hendricks SE, Weltin M. 1976. Effect of estrogen given during various periods of prepubertal life on the sexual behavior of rats Physiological Psychology 4, 105.
113. Mallampati RS, Johnson DC. 1974. Gonadotrophins in female rats androgenized by various treatments: prolactin as an index of hypothalamic damage. Neuroendocrinology 15, 255.
114. Whalen RE. 1968. Differentiation of the neural mechanisms which control gonadotrophin secretion and sexual behavior. In: Perspectives in reproduction and sexual behavior. Diamond M (ed). Bloomington: Indiana University Press.
115. Whalen RE, Nadler RD. 1963. Suppression of the development of female mating behavior by estrogen administration in infancy. Science 141: 273.
116. Brown-Grant K. 1973. Recent studies on the sexual differentiation of the brain. In: Foetal and neonatal physiology. Comline KS (ed). Cambridge: Cambridge University Press.
117. McDonald PG, Doughty C. 1973. Androgen sterilization in the neonatal female rat and its inhibition by an estrogen antagonist. Neuroendocrinology 13, 182.
118. McEwen BS. 1976. Steroid receptors in neuroendocrine tissue: topography, subcellular distribution and functional implications. In: Subcellular mechanisms in reproductive neuroendocrinology. Naftolin F, Ryan KJ, Davies J (eds). Amsterdam: Elsevier, p. 277.
119. Reddy VVR, Naftolin F, Ryan KJ. 1974. Conversion of androstenedione to estrone by neural tissues from fetal and neonatal rats. Endocrinology 94, 117.
120. Arai V. 1972. Effect of 5-dihydrotestosterone on differentiation of masculine pattern of the brain in the rat. Endocrinologica Japonica 19, 389.
121. Larsson K, Soedersten P, Beyer C. 1973. Sexual behavior in male rats treated with estrogen in combination with dihydrotestosterone. Hormones and Behavior 4, 289.
122. McDonald PG, Doughty C. 1974. Effect of neonatal administration of different androgens in the female rat: correlation between aromatization and the induction of sterilization. Journal of Endocrinology 61, 95.
123. Baum MJ, Vreeburg JTM. 1973. Copulation in castrated male rats following combined treatment with estradiol and dihydrotestosterone. Science 182, 283.
124. Naftolin F, Ryan KJ, Petro Z. 1972. Aromatization of androstenedione by the anterior hypothalamus of adult male and female rats. Endocrinology 90, 295.
125. Reddy VVR, Naftolin F, Ryan KJ. 1973. Aromatization in the central nervous system of rabbits: effects of castration and hormone treatment. Endocrinology 92, 589.
126. Weisz J, Gibbs C. 1974. Conversion of testosterone and androstenedione to estrogens in vitro by the brain of female rats. Endocrinology 94, 616.
127. Diamond M, Llacuna A, Wond CL. 1973. Sex behavior after neonatal progesterone, testosterone, estrogen or anti-androgens. Hormones and Behavior 4, 73.

128. Gray J, Levine S Broadhurst PL. 1965. Gonadal hormone injections in infancy and adult emotional behavior. Animal Behaviour 13, 33.
129. Schlenker G, Hinz G. 1974. Effect of prenatal treatment with testosterone oenanthate or oestradiol benzoate on gonadal function, sexual behavior, and growth of pigs. Archiv fuer Experimentelle Veterinarmedizin 28, 117.
130. Feder HH, Naftolin F, Ryan KJ. 1974. Male and female sexual responses in male rats given estradiol benzoate and 5alpha-androstan-17beta-ol-3one propionate. Endocrinology 94, 136.
131. Whalen RE, Battie C, Luttge WG. 1972. Anti-estrogen inhibition of androgen induced sexual receptivity in rats. Behavioral Biology 7, 311.
132. Soedersten P. 1974. Effects of an estrogen antagonist, MER-25, on mounting behavior and lordosis behavior in the female rat. Hormones and Behavior 5, 111.
133. Feder HH, Wade GN. 1974. Integrative actions of perinatal hormones on neural tissues mediating adult sexual behavior. In: The neurosciences: third study program. Schmitt FO, Worden FG (eds). Cambridge, Mass : MIT Press.
134. Greene RR, Burrill WJ, Ivy AC. 1939. Progesterone is androgenic. Endocrinology 24, 351.
135. McLaclan JA, Newbold RR. 1975. Reproductive tract lesions in male mice exposed prenatally to diethylstilbestrol. Science 190, 991.
136. Resko JA, Malley A, Begley D, Hess DL. 1973. Radioimmunoassay of testosterone during fetal development of the rhesus monkey. Endocrinology 93, 156.
137. Bloch E. 1964. Metabolism of 4-14C-progesterone by human fetal testes and ovaries. Endocrinology 74, 833.
138. Taylor T, Coutts JR, MacNaughton MC. 1974. Human foetal synthesis of testosterone from perfused progesterone. Journal of Endocrinology 60, 321.
139. Diez D'Aux RC, Murphy BEP. 1974. Androgens in the human fetus. Journal of Steroid Biochemistry 5, 207.
140. Reyes FI, Boroditsky RS, Winter JSD, Faiman C 1974. Studies on human sexual development. II. Fetal and maternal serum gonadotropin and sex steroid concentrations. Journal of Clinical Endocrinology and Metabolism 38, 612.
141. Abramovich RD. 1974. Human sexual differentiation - in utero influences. Journal of Obstetrics and Gynaecology of the British Commonwealth 81, 448.
142. Warne GL, Farman C, Reyes FI, Winter JS. 1977 Studies on human sexual development. V. Concentrations of testosterone, 17-hydroxyprogesterone and progesterone in human amniotic fluid throughout gestation Journal of Clinical Endocrinology and Metabolism 44, 934.
143. Robinson JD, Judd HL, Young PE, Jones OW, Yen SSC. 1977. Amniotic fluid androgens and estrogens in midgestation. Journal of Clinical Endocrinology and Metabolism 45, 755.

144. Doerner G, Stahl F, Rhode W, Robner P, Halle H, Schott G. 1975. Elevated free testosterone in the plasma of early pregnant women bearing male fetuses and of hypersexual men. Endokrinologie 65, 224.
145. Resko JA. 1975. Fetal hormones and their effect on the differentiation of the central nervous system in primates. Federation Proceedings 34, 1650.
146. Ehrhardt AA, Epstein R, Money J. 1968. Fetal androgens and female gender identity in the early-treated adrenogenital syndrome. Johns Hopkins Medical Journal 122, 160.
147. Ehrhardt AA, Evers K, Money J. 1968. Influence of androgen and some aspects of sexually dimorphic behavior in women with the late-treated adrenogenital syndrome. Johns Hopkins Medical Journal 123, 115.
148. Ehrhardt AA, Baker SW. 1974. Fetal androgens, human central nervous system differentiation, and behavioral sex differences. In: Sex differences in behavior. Friedman RC, Richart RM, Vande Wiele RL (eds). New York: Wiley, p. 33.
149. Ehrhardt AA Greenberg N, Money J. 1970. Female gender identity and absence of fetal gonadal hormones: Turner's syndrome. Johns Hopkins Medical Journal 126, 237.
150. Money J. 1965. Influence of hormones on sexual behavior. Annual Review of Medicine 16, 67.
151. Money J, Meredith T. 1967. Elevated verbal IQ and idiopathic precocious sexual maturation. Pediatric Research 1, 59.
152. Walker PA, Money J. 1972. Prenatal androgenization of females. Hormones 3, 119.
153. Masica DN, Money J, Ehrhardt AA, Lewis VG. 1969. IQ, fetal sex hormones and cognitive patterns: Studies in the testicular feminizing syndrome of androgen insensitivity. Johns Hopkins Medical Journal 124, 34.
154. Money J, Ehrhardt AA, Masica DN. 1968. Fetal feminization induced by androgen insensitivity in the testicular feminization syndrome: effect on marriage and maternalism. Johns Hopkins Medical Journal 123, 105.
155. Bongiovanni A, McPaddon A. 1960. Steroids during pregnancy and possible fetal consequences. Fertility and Sterility 11, 181.
156. Wilkins L. 1960. Masculinization of female fetus due to use of orally given progestins. Journal of The American Medical Association 172, 1028.
157. Burstein R, Wasserman HC. 1964. The effect of provera on the fetus. Obstetrics and Gynecology 23, 931.
158. Grumbach MM, Ducharme R. 1960. The effects of androgens on fetal sexual development: androgen-induced female pseudohermaphroditism. Fertility and Sterility 11, 157.
159. Grumbach MM, Ducharme R, Moloshok RE. 1959. On fetal masculinizing action of certain oral progestins. Journal of Clinical Endocrinology and Metabolism 19, 1369.

160. Hayles AB, Nolan RB. 1957. Female pseudohermaphroditism: report of case in an infant born of a mother receiving methyltestosterone during pregnancy. Proceedings of the Staff Meetings of the Mayo Clinic 32, 41.
161. Hayles AB, Nolan RB. 1958. Masculinization of female fetus, possibly related to administration of progesterone during pregnancy. Proceedings of the Staff Meetings of the Mayo Clinic 33, 200.
162. Jacobson BD. 1961. Abortion: its prediction and management. Clinical experience with norlutin. Fertility and Sterility 12, 474.
163. Jones HW, Wilkins L. 1960. The genital anomaly associated with prenatal exposure to progesterone. Fertility and Sterility 11, 148.
164. Wilkins L, Jones W, Holman G, Stempfel S. 1958. Masculinization of the female fetus associated with administration of oral and intramuscular progestins during gestation. Non-adrenal female pseudohermaphroditism. Journal of Clinical Endocrinology and Metabolism 18, 559.
165. Courrier R, Jost A. 1942. Intersexualité foetale provoquée par la pregnéninoline au cours de la grossesse. Comptes rendus des séances de la Société de biologie 136, 395.
166. Lerner LJ, Phillipo M, Yiacas E, Brennan D, Borman A. 1962. A comparison of the acetophenone derivatives of 16-17-dihydroprogesterone with other progestational steroids for masculinization of the rat fetus. Endocrinology 71, 448.
167. Neumann F, Graf KJ, Elger W. 1974. Hormone-induced disturbances in sexual differentiation. Advances in the Biosciences 13, 71.
168. Piotrowski J. 1968. Experimental investigations on the effect of progesterone on embryonal development. II. Investigation carried out on rabbits. Folia Biologica (Krakow) 16, 335.
169. Piotrowski J. 1968. The effect of progesterone on the foetal development of rats of the Wistar strain. Part III. Folia Biologica (Krakow) 16, 343.
170. Revesz C, Chappel CI, Gaudry R. 1960. Masculinization of female fetuses in the rat by progestational compounds. Endocrinology 66, 140.
171. Schoeler HFL, de Wachter AM. 1961. Evaluation of androgenic properties of progestational compounds in the rat by the female foetal masculinization test. Acta Endocrinologica 38, 128.
172. Suchowsky GK, Junkman K. 1961. A study of the virilizing effect of progestogens on the female rat fetus. Endocrinology 68, 341.
173. Whalen RE, Luttge WG. 1971. Differential localization of progesterone uptake in brain, role of sex, estrogen pretreatment and adrenalectomy. Brain Research 33, 147.
174. Whalen RE, Peck CK, LoPiccolo J. 1966. Virilization of female rats by prenatally administered progestin. Endocrinology 78, 965.

175. Chappell CI, Revesz C, Gauchy R. 1960. Biological studies on new orally active 6,17-halogenated progesterone. Acta Endocrinologica (Kbh) (suppl.) 51, 915.
176. Junkman K. 1963 Experimental aspects in the study of synthetic progestogens. Symposium of family planning Journal of the Egyptian Medical Association 38.
177. Kraay RJ, Brennan DM. 1963. Evaluation of chlormadione acetate and other progestins for foetal masculinization in rats. Acta Endocrinologica 43, 412.
178. Lerner LJ, Brennan DM, de Phillipo M, Yiacas E. 1961. Comparison of biological activities of progesterone, norethisterone, and the acetophenone derivatives of 16 alpha, 17 alpha-dihydroprogesterone. Federation Proceedings 20, 200.
179. Johnstone EE, Franklin RR. 1964. Assay of progestins for fetal virilization properties using the mouse. Obstetrics and Gynecology 23, 359.
180. Nora JJ, Nora AH, Blu J, Ingram J, Fountain A, Peterson M, Lortacher RH, Kimberling WJ. 1978. Exogenous progestogen and estrogen implicated in birth defects. Journal of the American Medical Association 240, 837.
181. Aarskog D. 1970. Clinical and cytogenetic studies in hypospadias. Acta Paediatrica Scandinavica (suppl.) 203, 1.
182. Aarskog D 1979. Maternal progestins as a possible cause of hypospadias. New England Journal of Medicine 300, 75.
183. Shapiro BH, Goldman AS, Bongiovanni AM, Marison JM. 1976. Neonatal progesterone and feminine sexual development. Nature 264, 795.
184. Hagemenas FC, Kittinger GW. 1972. The influence of fetal sex on plasma progesterone levels. Endocrinology 91, 253.
185. McDonald GJ, Yoshinaga K, Greep RO. 1973. Serum progesterone values in macaca mulatta near term. American Journal of Physical Anthropology 38, 201.
186. Cagnoni M, Fantini F, Morace G, Ghetti A. 1965. Failure of testosterone propionate to induce the 'early androgen' syndrome in rats previously injected with progesterone. Journal of Endocrinology 33, 527.
187. Kincl FA, Maqueo M. 1965. Prevention of steroid-induced sterility in neonatal male and female rats. Endocrinology 77, 859.
188. Heinonen OP, Sloane D, Monson RR, Hook EB, Shapiro S. 1977. Cardiovascular birth defects and antenatal exposure to female sex hormones. New England Journal of Medicine 296, 67.
189. Heinonen OP, Sloane D, Shapiro S. 1977. Hormones, hormone antagonists and contraceptives: birth defects and drugs in pregnancy. Littleton: Publishing Sciences Group, p 338.
190. Dalton K. 1968. Ante-natal progesterone and intelligence. British Journal of Psychiatry 114, 1377.
191. Reinisch JM, Karow WG. 1977. Prenatal exposure to synthetic progestins and estrogens: effects on human development. Archives of Sexual Behavior 6, 257.

192. Meyer-Bahlburg HFL, Grisanti GC, Ehrhardt AA. 1977. Perinatal effects of sex hormones on human male behavior: Medroxyprogesterone acetate (MPA). Psychoneuroendocrinology 2, 383.
193. Ambani LM, Joshi NJ, Vardija RA, Devi PK. 1977. Are hormonal contraceptives teratogenic? Fertility and Sterility 28, 791.
194. Ehrhardt AA, Money J. 1967. Progestin-induced hermaphroditism: IQ and psychosexual identity in a study of ten girls. Journal of Sex Research 3, 83.
195. Campbell DT, Stanley JC. 1963. Experimental and quasi-experimental designs for research. Chicago: Rand McNally.
196. Dalton K. 1976. Prenatal progesterone and educational attainments. British Journal of Psychiatry 129, 433.
197. Zussman JU, Zussman PP, Dalton K. 1975. Post-pubertal effects of prenatal administration of progesterone. Paper presented at the Meeting of the Society for Research in Child Development. Denver.
198. Lynch A, Mychalkim W, Hutt SJ. 1978. Prenatal progesterone. I. Its effect on development and on intellectual and academic achievement. Early Human Development 2, 305.
199. Ehrhardt AA, Grisanti GC, Meyer-Bahlburg HFL. 1977. Prenatal exposure to medroxyprogesterone acetate (MPA) in girls. Psychoneuroendocrinology 2, 391.
200. Reinisch JM. 1977. Prenatal exposure of human foetuses to synthetic progestin and oestrogen affects personality Nature 266, 561.
201. Cattell RB, Eber HW, Maurice M. 1970. Handbook for sixteen personality factor questionnaires. Champaign, Illinois: Institute for Personality and Ability Testing.
202. Reinisch JM. 1979. Prenatal hormone exposure and aggressive response in humans Mexico City: Fifth world congress of sexology.
203. Leifer AD, Roberts DF. 1971. Children's responses to television violence. Stanford: Institute for Communication Research.
204. Jick HR. 1975. What to expect from prednisone. Drug Therapy 5, 85.
205. DeCosta EJ, Ableman MA. 1952. Cortisone and pregnancy: an experimental and clinical study of the effects of cortisone on gestation. American Journal of Obstetrics and Gynecology 64, 746.
206. Kenny FM, Preeyasombat C, Spaulding JS, Migeon CJ. 1966. Cortisol production rate. IV. Infants born of steroid-treated mothers and of diabetic mothers Infants with trisomy syndrome and with anencephaly. Pediatrics 37, 960.
207. Margulis RR, Hodgkinson CP. 1953. Evaluation of the safety of corticotropin (ACTH) and cortisone in pregnancy. Obstetrics and Gynecology 1, 276.

208. Schatz M, Patterson R, Zeitz S, O'Rourke J, Melam H. 1975. Corticosteroid therapy for the pregnant asthmatic patient. Journal of the American Medical Association 233, 804.
209. Walsh SD, Clark FR. Pregnancy in patients on long-term corticosteroid therapy Scottish Medical Journal 12, 302.
210. Warrell DW, Taylor R. 1968. Outcome for the foetus of mothers receiving prednisone during pregnancy Lancet 1, 117.
211. Yackel DB, Kembers RD, McConahey WM. 1966. Adreno-corticosteroid therapy in pregnancy. American Journal of Obstetrics and Gynecology 96, 985.
212. Greenblatt RB, Barfield WE, Lampros CP. 1956. Cortisone in the treatment of infertility Fertility and Sterility 7, 203.
213. Jeffries WMcK, Levy RP. 1959. Treatment of ovarian dysfunction with small doses of cortisone or hydrocortisone. Journal of Clinical Endocrinology and Metabolism 19, 1069.
214. Jeffries WMcK, Weir WC, Weir DR, Prouty RL. 1958. The use of cortisone and related steroids in infertility. Fertility and Sterility 9, 145.
215. Reinisch JM, Gandelman R. 1978. Human research in behavioral endocrinology: methodological and theoretical considerations. In: Hormones and brain development. Doerner G, Kawakami M (eds). Amsterdam: Elsevier, p.77.
216. Besedovsky HO. 1974. Suppression of fetal hemotopoetic development by prednisone treatment of pregnant rats. Experientia 15, 1098.
217. Blackburn WR, Kaplan HS. 1963. Effects of prednisolone on the developing rat fetus with special reference to the thymus Federation Proceedings 22, 601.
218. Blackburn WR, Kaplan HS, McKay DG. 1965. Morphologic changes in the developing rat placenta following prednisolone administration. American Journal of Obstetrics and Gynecology 92, 234.
219. Frasier CF, Feinstat TD. 1951. Production of congenital defects in the offspring of pregnant mice treated with cortisone. Pediatrics 8, 527.
220. Glauback S, Antopol W, Graff S. 1951. Excessive doses of cortisone in pregnant mice: effect on development and survival of the fetus and newborn and on the maternal breast tissue. Bulletin of the New York Academy of Sciences 27, 358.
221. Karnofsky DA, Stock CC, Rhoads CP. 1950. The effect of adrenal steroids on growth of chick embryo. Federation Proceedings 9, 290.
222. Karnofsky DA, Ridgway LP, Patterson PA. 1951. Growth-inhibiting effect of cortisone acetate on the chick embryo. Endocrinology 48, 596.
223. Karnofsky DA, Ridgway LP, Stock CC. 1951. Growth inhibition by cortisone and related steroids. Federation Proceedings 10, 204.
224. Reinisch JM, Simon NG, Karow WG, Gandelman R. 1978. Prenatal prednisone exposure in humans and animals retards intrauterine growth. Science 202, 436.

225. Beitins IZ, Bayard F, Ances IG, Kowarski A, Migeon CJ. 1972. The transplacental passage of prednisone and prednisolone in pregnancy near term. Journal of Pediatrics 81, 936.
226. Beitins IZ, Bayard F, Ances IG, Kowarski A, Migeon CJ. 1973. The metabolic clearance rate, blood production, interconversion and transplacental passage of cortisol and cortisone in pregnancy near term. Pediatric Research 7, 509.
227. Migeon CJ, Bertrand J, Gemzell CA. 1961. The transplacental passage of various steroid hormones in mid-pregnancy. Recent Progress in Hormone Research 17, 207.
228. Migeon CJ, Prystowsky H, Grumbach MM, Byron MC. 1956. Placental passage of 17-hydroxycorticosteroids comparison of the levels in maternal and fetal plasma and effect of ACTH and hydrocortisone administration. Journal of Clinical Investigation 35, 488.
229. Zarrow MX, Philpot JE, Denenberg V. 1970. Passage of ^{14}C-4-corticosterone from the rat mother to the fetus and neonate. Nature 226, 1058.
230. Reimer LG, Morris HG, Ellis EF. 1975. Growth of asthmatic children during treatment with alternate-day steroids. Journal of Allergy and Clinical Immunology 55, 224.
231. Gunberg DL. 1957. Some effects of exogenous hydrocortisone on pregnancy in the rat. Anatomical Record 129, 133.
232. Neligan GA. 1967. The clinical effects of being 'light for dates'. Sec. Obstet. Gynaec. 60, 881.
233. McBurney RD. 1947. The undernourished full-term infant: a case report. The Western Journal of Surgery, Obstetrics and Gynecology 55, 363.
234. World Health Organization. 1961. Expert Committee on Maternal and Child Health. WHO Technical Report Series 217.
235. Babson SG, Kangas J, Young N, Bramhall JL. 1964. Growth and development of twins of dissimilar size at birth. Pediatrics 33, 327
236. Elliott K, Knight J (eds). 1974. Size at birth Ciba Foundation Symposium 27 (new series). Amsterdam: Associated Scientific Publishers
237. Fitzhardinge PM, Steven EM. 1972. The small-for-date infant. I. Later growth patterns. Pediatrics 49, 671.
238. Fitzhardinge PM, Steven EM. 1972. The small-for-date infant. II. Pediatrics 50, 50.
239. Gruenwald P. 1962. Full-term and low birth weight. Pediatrics 29, 333.
240. Sinclair JC, Coldiron JS. 1969. Low birthweight and postnatal physical development. Developmental Medicine and Child Neurology 11, 314.
241. Walker J. 1967. The 'small for dates' baby. Sec. Obstet Gynaec 60:877.
242. Reinisch JM, Simon NG, Gandelman R. 1980. Prenatal exposure to prednisone permanently alters fighting behavior of female mice. Pharmacology, Biochemistry and Behavior 12, 213.

243. vom Saal FS. 1976. Prenatal androgen and aggression in mice. Newark, New Jersey: Rutgers University, unpublished doctoral dissertation.
244. Simon NG, Gandelman R. 1977. Decreased aggressive behavior in the offspring of ACTH-treated mice. Behavioral Biology 21, 478.
245. Ward I. 1977. Exogenous androgen activates female behavior in noncopulating, prenatally stressed male rats. Journal of Comparative and Physiological Psychology 91, 465.
246. Broulik PD, Starka L. 1975. Corticosteroid-like effect of cyproterone and cyproterone acetate in mice. Experientia 31, 1364.
247. Svare BB, Gandelman R. 1976. Suckling stimulation induces aggression in virgin female mice. Nature 260, 606.
248. Lynch A, Mychalkim W. 1978. Prenatal progesterone. II. Its role in the treatment of pre-eclamptic toxaemia and its effect on the offspring's intelligence: a reappraisal. Early Human Development 2, 323.
249. McMahon FG. 1974. Corticosteroids in clinical practice American Family Physician 10, 132.
250. Neumann F, Steinbeck H. 1972. Influence of sexual hormones on the differentiation of neural centers. Archives of Sexual Behavior 2, 147.
251. Ward IL. 1972. Female sexual behavior in male rats treated prenatally with an anti-androgen. Physiology and Behavior 8, 53.
252. Ward IL. 1974. Sexual behavior differentiation: prenatal hormonal and environmental control. In: Sex differences in behavior Friedman RC, Richart RM, Vande Wiele RL (eds). New York: Wiley.

6. THE EFFECTS OF A CHRONIC ILLNESS ON SOMATIC GROWTH AND PSYCHOLOGICAL DEVELOPMENT

G. SINNEMA

INTRODUCTION

There is no doubt that a chronic illness can have a profound influence on both the somatic growth and the psychological development of children and adolescents. Diseases such as diabetes mellitus, asthma, congenital heart disease, chronic renal failure and cystic fibrosis can all cause a slowing down of somatic growth and maturation. 'The actual mechanisms whereby growth is slowed probably vary at least somewhat from one disease to another' (1). In some cases growth retardation is due to medication (e.g. corticosteroids). Discussion of physiological factors responsible for growth retardation is beyond the scope of this paper. These factors have been recently reviewed by Van den Brande and Rappaport (2).

Psychological development -social, emotional and cognitive- may be delayed or disturbed. After reviewing the literature on this subject, we shall report on a recent research-project on the delay in growth and development of adolescents with cystic fibrosis. This project is being carried out in the University Children's Hospital in Utrecht.

REVIEW OF THE LITERATURE

Generally, a chronic illness is regarded as a non-specific source of stress affecting the psychological and social development of the child and the adolescent (3). Whether or not this stress leads to a disturbance of normal development depends more on factors such as the personality of the child, patterns of interaction within the family, and attitudes within the society than on the severity and the specific somatic characteristics of the disease. The hypothesis of non-specificity implies that there is no such thing as a 'diabetic' or 'asthmatic' type of personality (4). Although there is no 'disease-specificity', there is some evidence that the curability of a disease and the moment of onset of symptoms have a bearing on the degree to which a chronic disease affects psychological development (5).

Many problems arise in connection with chronically ill children and adolescents The literature up to 1975 has been reviewed by Pless and Pinkterton (6). Physically ill children are often found to be socially maladjusted or isolated. They tend to be more anxious and to have lower self-esteem than healthy children. Many studies demonstrate that chronically ill children have a distorted body image, especially in adolescence. Overprotection by parents may cause a delay in a child's personality development ('immaturity'). 'Yet', to cite Tavormina (7), 'since most studies in the current literature were based on assumptions, clinical impressions, subjective evaluations, or abbreviated projective techniques, the findings should be considered tentative and largely speculative'.

Epidemiològical research is much less impressive, especially as regards quantity. In three extensive health-surveys chronically ill children and adolescents were shown to have more psychological, psychiatric and social problems than their healthy peers (8). A recent review of these studies can be found in Roghmann (9). Experimental research, using control-groups, is relatively scarce. The fact that controlled studies often pertain to specific clinical populations makes conclusions about psychological abnormality somewhat suspect. In contrast to the results of these studies and to the 'impressionistic' literature, the more systematic studies often report that the psychological development of chronically ill children and adolescents is essentially normal (7,10,11,12). However, even these 'better' studies may suffer from methodological shortcomings. For instance, the recent findings of Zeltzer et al. (12), who assert the 'essentially healthy psychological status of chronically ill adolescents', are based on a very short illness-impact questionnaire. The questionnaire was self-administered, partially in a group situation. The authors admit that the psychological mechanism of denial could have seriously affected their results. They then point to the adaptational value of denial. They may be correct about this, but it weakens their conclusions about psychological normality.

The cognitive development of chronically ill adolescents, as measured by I.Q. or by scholastic achievement, is found to be quite normal in some studies (13), retarded in others (14). Some authors claim that chronically ill children have a superior level of (verbal) intelligence (15,16). This is explained by the hypothesis of psychological compensation: physical weakness leads to accentuation of cognitive development. However, population studies generally fail to demonstrate the prevalence of superior intelligence in chronically ill children (17).

Retardation of somatic growth can in itself have effects on psychological development. Findings in the literature are comparable to those concerning the effects of chronic illness. 'Adolescents with growth and sexual retardation suffer from social, emotional and scholastic problems' (18). Examples of social problems are: 'difficulties in interrelationship with the other sex; a tendency to have much younger friends; avoidance of social activities; still being called 'boy' or 'girl' (...) in late adolescence; boys - sometimes being approached as girls by strangers' (18). Emotional problems are connected with the establishment of sexual identity and a stable body image, and with emotional lability (e.g. depression).

Reports in the literature about the effects of small stature and delayed puberty due to chronic illness resemble reports in the literature about the effects of early and late maturation. In a review article, Gross and Duke (19) conclude that late maturing boys, as compared to early maturing boys, are generally disadvantaged in their social and psychological development. Even as adults they are less popular and have lower occupational status. For girls the situation seems to be more complicated, but less is known about female development. It should be noted that the interpretation of differences between early and late maturing adolescents depends somewhat on normative values about personality. Whereas early maturing boys are more sociable, more enterprising and more goal-directed, they are also less flexible and less reflective than late maturing boys. The evaluation of these characteristics varies with the cultural context (20). Furthermore, there is some danger in extrapolating the results of the maturation-studies to the study of chronic illness. Early and late maturation, as well as the behavioural correlates, may be due to one common factor (e.g. a genetic one), whereas in chronic illness there is a complex interaction between the illness, retarded growth, maturation and psychological development.

CYSTIC FIBROSIS

A research-project on adolescent growth and development

Cystic fibrosis is an example of a chronic illness that has marked effects on somatic growth and maturation, as well as on psychological development. Cystic fibrosis (CF) is the most common lethal genetic disease among children of Caucasian populations. It is assumed to be a metabolic disease, although the basic defect is unknown. The median life expectancy for patients with CF is about 19 years, at least in some centres in the United States (21). The incidence in The Netherlands has been estimated to be 1 in 3600 (22). Chronic obstructive pulmonary disease and pancreatic insufficiency with malabsorption are the major clinical manifestations. Treatment is symptomatic. Malabsorption is controlled with oral pancreatic enzymes. In order to prevent pulmonary infections, patients are given chest percussion, postural drainage and breathing exercises. Antibiotics are used to treat acute infections, but at a more advanced stage of the disease antibiotics are often prescribed continuously.

Our research-project on the somatic growth and the psychological development of adolescents with CF consists of 3 separate parts, proceeding from a more general to a more specific level of analysis: 1) an epidemiological survey, aimed at giving an overall picture of the delay or deviance in growth and development; 2) a comparative study on the establishment of independence in four groups of adolescents: adolescents with CF, adolescents with asthma, healthy adolescents with small stature and delayed puberty, and healthy control adolescents. In this paper we shall report on the design and on some results of these first two studies. The aim of the third part of the project, 3), is to find out whether delay or deviance in psychological development is functional or dysfunctional in coping with the disease. We intend to do this by analysing in depth the longitudinal case-histories of selected CF-patients. On this level the role of the psychological mechanisms of denial will be given special attention. We shall report on this part of the study in a later publication.

Adolescents with CF in The Netherlands: a survey

The CF population

In 1979 nearly all 489 Dutch paediatricians and 369 chest physicians were asked to fill in a short questionnaire for every patient, born before 1971, and currently under their care. The ultimate response was 96%. The number of patients was 309, with an age-range of 8-40 years (table 1). The younger and older age groups were included to get a better understanding of trends during adolescence (ages: 12-20 years). There were more male patients (57%) than female patients (43%, $p<.05$); the corresponding figures in the general population are 51 and 49. In the following the figures for the Dutch population as a whole are based on the most recent data that could be obtained on request from the Netherlands Central Bureau of Statistics.

Table 1. Number of cystic fibrosis patients in The Netherlands born before 1.1.1971 according to age and sex (figures for 1979).

Age (y)	Male patients	Female patients	Total
8- 9	29	20	49
10-11	24 (52%)	29 (48%)	53 (100%)
12-13	38	20	58
14-15	25	20	45
16-17	27 (61%)	17 (39%)	44 (100%)
18-19	10	9	19
20-21	7	6	13
22-23	5	5	10
24-40	10 (53%)	8 (47%)	18 (100%)
8-40	175 (57%)	134 (43%)	309 (100%)

The age group 12-17 years was especially dominated by boys (61%); in the age group 12-13 years the figure was as high as 66! Whereas the higher mortality in females with CF is well documented in the literature (22,23,24), it is not quite clear why this higher mortality occurs during early adolescence. Gurwitz et al. (21) mention the possible role of hormonal as well as psychological factors.

Somatic growth: height and weight

Retarded growth in patients with CF is probably correlated with pulmonary and gastro-intestinal dysfunctions (2,25,26). Skeletal maturity and onset of puberty (growth spurt; sexual maturity) are delayed in the majority of male and female CF-patients (27,28). The mean height of all patients is below the population mean, but the distribution is fairly normal (29). Generally, gain in weight is more severely affected than gain in height, especially in females (29).

For our survey we used the most recent data available on height and weight. For every patient, height in centimetres was transformed into a standard deviation score (SDSH), using the Dutch reference values of van Wieringen (30). The height of 73% of CF-patients appears to be below the mean for age. Boys are on average more retarded than girls ($p<.01$). The mean height for boys is about 6 cm below normal, for girls about 3 cm. The sex difference in SDSH may, at least partially, be due to pubertal delay in both sexes. This would mean a maximal discrepancy when healthy adolescents are going into the pubertal spurt. Hence the drop in SDSH is shown earlier in girls than in boys.

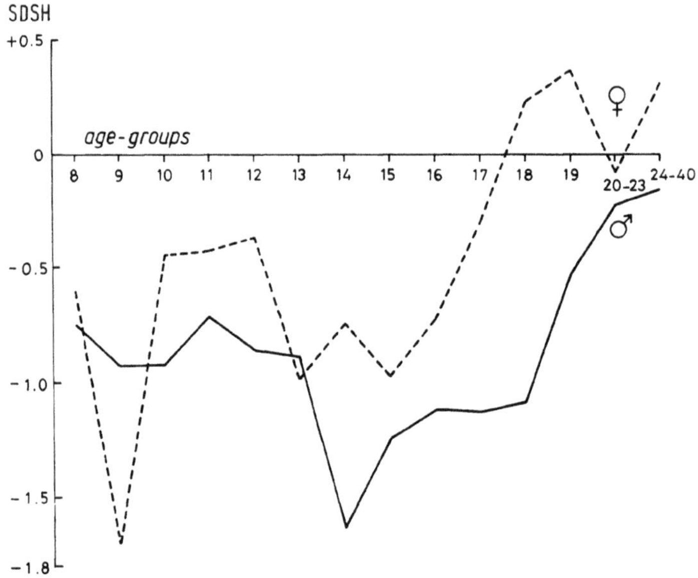

Figure 1. Cystic fibrosis patients in 1979 (n=295): average standard deviation scores for height (SDSH) according to sex and age group

Figure 1 shows the average SDSH according to sex and age group. Except for the groups aged 9 (n=6) and 13 years, the mean values for girls are higher than those for boys. Male patients older than 20 years, and female patients older than 17 years show little deviation from the normal values. This is in agreement with the conclusion of Mearns (31), namely that CF-patients can achieve the same adult height as healthy children, provided the disease follows a relatively favourable course.

Weight in kgs has been transformed into a percentile category, according to height, sex and age, using the reference values of van Wieringen (30). Weight for height is below P10 in 54% of patients; only in 15% it is above the median. Decrease in weight with age is most pronounced in males: the percentage below P10 rises from 37 between 8 and 11 years to 50 between 12 and 17, and to 91 in the 18 and above age group. For girls the corresponding figures are 54, 56 and 62%. The data on weight for height have been further elaborated by expressing every individual weight for height as a percentage of the corresponding

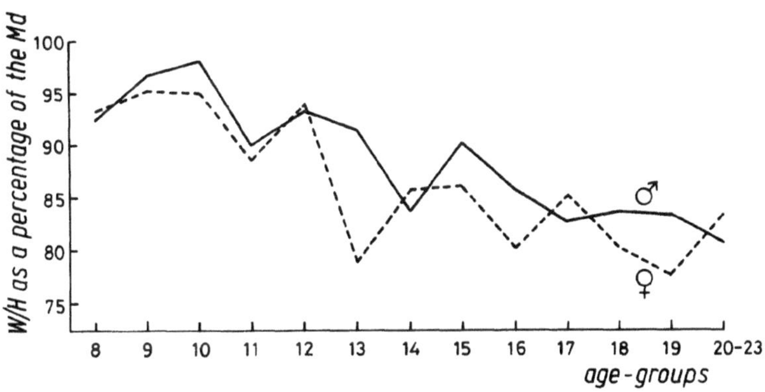

Figure 2. Cystic fibrosis patients in 1979 (n=282): averages for weight in relation to height (W/H), expressed as a percentage of the median normal value (Md) according to sex and age group. Since there are so few patients aged between 24 and 40 this group has been omitted.

median normal value. Figure 2 shows the mean percentages according to sex and age group. Mean weight for height is lower in girls than in boys ($p<.05$). Whereas for the older patients height increases (figure 1), weight for height decreases. This combination of findings probably expresses a late growth spurt in height, without a corresponding increase in weight. The decrease of weight for height with age reflects the progressive nature of the disease. Weight for height is a more accurate indication of the degree of deterioration in CF than height (32).

Psychological development: self-support, education and vocation

One of the major developmental tasks of adolescence is the establishment of independence; this is generally assumed to be a very difficult task for the adolescent with CF. Most authors stress the importance of guidance and counselling. There are only a few epidemiological surveys that contain information about the development of independence (33,34).

In our survey we looked at some simple parameters for the development of independence: 1) self-support: living with parents versus living alone or with a permanent partner; 2) education: primary versus secondary school; education versus employment; general versus vocational education.

The results indicate that adolescents and young adults with CF do not stay longer than normal in the protective environment of their home. The majority of patients (90%) in the 15-19 age group (n=85) live at home with their parents; the corresponding figure in the total population of The Netherlands is 92%. In the 20-24 age group (n=25) 14 patients (56%) still live with their parents; the corresponding figure in the total population is 54%. Of the 13 men with CF who have left home, 6 are married or living with a permanent partner; of the 19 women who no longer live with their parents, 8 are married or living with a partner.

CF-patients usually leave primary school somewhat later than their normal peers. The percentage of 12 to 14-year-olds who are still receiving (normal) primary education is 1.5 times as high as in the population as a whole.

Almost all older adolescents with CF are still receiving some form of education. In the 16-20 age group 90% of the boys and 69% of the girls attend day-school full-time; the corresponding figures in the general population are 49% and 34% respectively ($p<.001$). In the 16-40 age group (n=104) only 35 patients (13 men, 22 women) are no longer receiving education. Sixteen patients are living on a social security allowance. Only 19 patients (5 men, 14 women) are working. The word 'working' is used in a very liberal sense and includes for instance all kinds of part-time work. Among the jobs being held by CF-patients are receptionist, secretary, sales assistant, civil servant, assistant manager in a supermarket.

The fact that CF-patients spend more years in the educational system may indicate slow development and lack of progress in school. But it may also reflect the tendency of many parents and paediatricians to keep patients in the educational system, which is a relatively protective environment compared to the competitive aspects of the labour-market. It is not surprising, therefore, that the percentage of CF-patients receiving general education is higher than the percentage receiving vocational training. This is also true of normal adolescents. In the case of CF-patients however, the percentage receiving general education is much higher. In the 12-20 age group 70% of male CF-patients receive general education and 30% vocational training, compared with 54% and 46% in the population as a whole ($p<.01$). For the girls these figures are for the CF-group 76% (general education) and 24% (vocational training) and for the normal population 61% and 39% ($p<.10$). Eight patients are at University; 6 patients are receiving higher vocational training.

Our data on self-support, education and employment of adolescents with CF, only partly support the hypothesis of a delay in social development. On the level of self-concept and adaptation to the illness, these data can be seen as providing the social context in which the development of independence takes place.

The development of independence: a closer look

In the second part of our research-project, the concept of CF is considered to be made up of three major elements: 1) the chronic nature; 2) the fatal outcome of the illness; and 3) the visibility of the handicap (retarded growth). In order to study the influence of these 'organismic' variables on adolescent independence, a semi-experimental design has been set up. Besides the CF-group, three reference groups have been chosen: a group of adolescents with asthma (chronic, but not fatal), a group of healthy, but small adolescents, and a group of 'normal', healthy controls The illness groups as such will be divided into a group of normal stature (height between P25 and P75), and one of small stature (height below P25).

Independence, as perceived by the adolescent, is being measured by an extensive questionnaire, filled in by a trained interviewer in a semi-structured interview. The interview has the character of a private, confidential talk; for that purpose, questions with open-ended answers have been mixed with questions with precoded answers. Only the latter are crucial in our measurement of independence. Generally, the alternatives form a 5-point-scale, indicating degrees of independence. Summing up of scores on separate questions leads to scoring (0-6) on the variables of independence (table 2). As an illustration, a question is given for the variable 'rules about health'. Question: who sees that you get enough sleep? Answers: 1) always my father/mother; 2) mostly my father/mother; 3) sometimes my father/mother looks after it, sometimes I do; 4) mostly I do; 5) always I do. Besides independence, some other relevant factors are measured: cognitive development; emotional support; body attitude; optimism/pessimism about the future and attitudes about illness. The physician scores the severity of the illness (35) and the extent and type of treatment. Somatic growth is evaluated by height, weight, and the stage of puberty. So far, data are available for 30 adolescents with CF (mean age 15.5 years), 58 healthy control adolescents (mean age 14.8 years) and 14 healthy controls with small stature (mean age 14.9 years; height below P25). As all groups are still being extended, only a few preliminary results are presented here, as an illustration of the type of data this level of analysis will provide.

In figure 3 the results on the eight variables of independence are presented. Generally, CF-patients show a delay in the development of intimacy/sexuality. This applies especially to the boys. Compared with their healthy peers, boys with CF are less interested in the other sex, and less often have (had) a girl friend. The delay in the development of intimacy/sexuality corresponds with the delay in the onset of puberty (oigarche;

Table 2. Variables in the development of independence.

1. Intimacy/sexuality (IS)
2. Body hygiene (BH)
3. Rules about health (HR)
4. Range of social activities (SA)
5. Management of conflicts (MC)
6. Planning own affairs (OA)
7. Opinions about politics, religion and ethics (PRE)
8. Ideals/ambitions (IA)

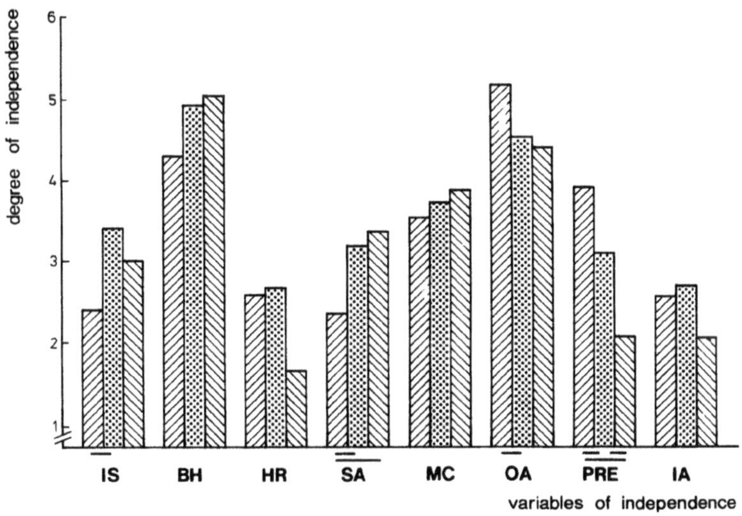

Figure 3. The development of independence for three groups of adolescents: patients with cystic fibrosis (n=30; at the left); healthy controls (n=58; in the middle); healthy adolescents with small stature (n=14; at the right). Underlining indicates statistical significance (p<.05).

menarche). Puberty has begun in 43% of CF-patients, in 88% of the healthy adolescents, and in 50% of the healthy, small adolescents. CF-patients appear to have fewer social activities outside the home - not surprising in the light of their physical handicap. However, in planning their own affairs (e.g. responsibility for doing their homework) CF-patients appear to be somewhat more independent than their healthy peers. CF-patients show more interest in politics, religion and ethics ('What is wrong or right in the world'), and have clearer opinions about these matters. The cognitive development of the CF-patients is superior to that of the healthy adolescents (mean I.Q. for the CF-group: 120.3; for the healthy controls: 109.5; for the small stature group: 99.9). CF-patients have more optimistic expectations about personal happiness in the future, in spite of possible set-backs.

DISCUSSION

The results of the population-survey indicate that there is some delay in the social development of adolescents and young adults with CF. For instance, they stay longer than their healthy peers in the protective environment of the school. However, the danger of extrapolating these findings to the psychological development of the adolescent is clearly demonstrated by the preliminary results of the second part of our study. There is no such thing as a general 'immaturity' in the development of independence Adolescents with CF do not differ from healthy adolescents as regards responsibility for body hygiene and health rules, management of conflicts, and formation of ideals and ambitions. CF-patients do have fewer social activities outside the home, probably due to their restricted physical capacities. Corresponding with a later onset of puberty, the adolescent with CF shows a delay in the development of intimacy and sexuality. However, the chronically ill adolescents are superior to their healthy peers as regards cognitive development, interest in politics, religion and ethics, and planning their own affairs.

The results of the comparative study should be regarded as hypotheses which will have to be tested in the forthcoming definitive analysis. If confirmed, the findings will certainly have a bearing on clinical practice. It is clear that general labels such as 'independent' or 'immature' are of little use. It will be necessary to differentiate between several types of independence, since a patient may function at a different level for each type.

To conlude, by considering psychologically relevant components of the concept of chronic illness such as its chronicity, its visibility and its fatal outcome, and by measuring the influence of these components on the development of different types of independence, we can obtain a broader and more detailed understanding of the psychological development of chronically ill adolescents.

ACKNOWLEDGEMENT

The author is grateful for the assistance he received from J.V.L. van den Brande, Professor of Paediatrics, J.W. Stoop, Professor of Paediatrics, J.C.J. Bonarius, Professor of Personality Psychology.

REFERENCES

1. Tanner JM. 1962. Growth at adolescence. Oxford: Blackwell.
2. van den Brande JL, Rappaport R. 1982. Croissance normale et ses déviations. In: Traité d'endocrinologie pédiatrique. Bertrand J, Rappaport R, Sizonenko PC (eds). Lausanne: Payot.
3. Korsch BM. 1973. Effect of chronic illness on adolescents and young adults. In: Fundamental problems of cystic fibrosis and related diseases. Mangos JA, Talamo RC (eds). New York: Intercontinental Medical Book Corporation.
4. Greydanus DE, Hofmann AD. 1979. Psychological factors in diabetes mellitus. American Journal of Diseases of Children 133, 1061.
5. Appelboom-Fondu J. 1978. Correlation between the age of onset of a chronic illness and the child's psychological adaptation to it. In: Auxology: human growth in health and disorder. Gedda L, Parisi P (eds). London: Academic Press.
6. Pless IB, Pinkterton P. 1975. Chronic childhood disorder. London: Henry Kimpton Publishers.
7. Tavormina JB, Kastner LS, Slater PM, Watt SL. 1976. Chronically ill children. A psychologically and emotionally deviant population? Journal of Abnormal Child Psychology 4, 99.
8. Pless IB, Roghmann KJ. 1971. Chronic illness and its consequences: observations based on three epidemiologic surveys. Journal of Pediatrics 79, 351.
9. Roghmann KJ. 1981. Die Familie als Patient: zum Wandel des Krankheitsbegriffs der Paediatrie in der Betreuung chronisch kranker Kinder. In: Chronisch kranke Kinder und Jugendliche in der Familie. Angermeyer MC, Doehner O (eds). Stuttgart: Enke Verlag.
10. Gayton WF, Friedman SB, Tavormina JB, Tucker F. 1977. Children with cystic fibrosis. Psychological test findings of patients, siblings and parents. Pediatrics 59, 888.
11. Kellerman J, Zeltzer L, Ellenberg L, Dash J, Rigler D. 1980. Psychological effects of illness in adolescence. Anxiety, self-esteem, and perception of control. Journal of Pediatrics 97, 126.
12. Zeltzer L, Kellerman J, Elleberg L, Dash J, Rigler D. 1980. Psychological effects of illness in adolescence. Impact of illness in adolescents - crucial issues and coping styles. Journal of Pediatrics 97, 132.
13. Cytryn L, van Moore P, Robinson ME. 1973. Psychological adjustment of children with cystic fibrosis. In: The child in his family. The impact of disease and death. Anthony EJ, Koupernik C (eds). New York: Wiley.
14. Burton L. 1975. The family life of sick children. London: Routledge and Kegan Paul.
15. Lawler RH, Nakielny W, Wright NA. 1966. Psychological implications of cystic fibrosis. Canadian Medical Association Journal 94, 1043.

16. Boyle IR, di Sant'Agnese PA, Sack S, Millican F, Kulczycki LL. 1976. Emotional adjustment of adolescents and young adults with cystic fibrosis. Journal of Pediatrics 88, 318.
17. Falkman C. 1977. Cystic fibrosis. A psychological study of 52 children and their families. Acta Paediatrica Scandinavica (suppl.) 269, 1.
18. Galatzer A, Rosenblith E, Laron Z. 1978. Psychological and rehabilitation aspects of short stature and delayed puberty. In: Auxology: human growth in health and disorder. Gedda L, Parisi P (eds). London: Academic Press.
19. Gross RT, Duke PM. 1980. The effect of early versus late physical maturation on adolescent behaviour. Pediatric Clinics of North America 27, 71.
20. de Wit J, van der Veer G. 1977. Psychologie van de adolescentie. Nijkerk: Callenbach.
21. Gurwitz D, Corey M, Francis PWJ, Crozier D, Levison H. 1979. Perspectives in cystic fibrosis. Pediatric Clinics of North America 26, 603.
22. ten Kate LP. 1977. Cystic fibrosis in The Netherlands. International Journal of Epidemiology 6, 23.
23. Warwick WJ, Pogue RE, Gerber HU, Nesbitt CJ. 1975. Survival patterns in cystic fibrosis. Journal of Chronic Diseases 28, 609.
24. Wood RE, Boat TF, Doershuk CF. 1976. Cystic fibrosis, state of the art. American Review of Respiratory Diseases 113, 833.
25. Sproul A, Huang N. 1964. Growth patterns in children with cystic fibrosis. Journal of Pediatrics 65, 664.
26. Kreissl T, Bender SW, Moerchen R, Hoevels O. 1972. The physical development of children with cystic fibrosis. Zeitschrift fuer Kinderheilkunde 113, 93.
27. Mitchell-Heggs P, Mearns M, Batten JC. 1976. Cystic fibrosis in adolescents and adults. Quarterly Journal of Medicine 45, 479.
28. Batten J. 1980. Clinical management of the adolescent and adult patient. In: Perspectives in cystic fibrosis. Sturgess JM (ed). Toronto: Canadian CF Foundation.
29. Corey ML. 1980. Longitudinal studies in cystic fibrosis. In: Perspectives in cystic fibrosis. Sturgess JM (ed). Toronto: Canadian CF Foundation.
30. van Wieringen JC. 1972. Secular changes of growth (review, tables and graphs), 1964-1966 height and weight surveys in The Netherlands in historical perspective. Leiden: Netherlands Institute for Preventive Medicine TNO.
31. Mearns MB. 1980. The heights of CF patients aged 2-9 years allowing for parental height and severity of pulmonary episodes from birth. In: Perspectives in cystic fibrosis. Sturgess JM (ed). Toronto: Canadian CF Foundation.
32. Dodge JA, Yassa JG. 1980. Food intake and supplementary feeding programmes. In: Perspectives in cystic fibrosis. Sturgess JM (ed). Toronto: Canadian CF Foundation.
33. Shwachmann H, Kowalski M, Khaw K-T. 1977. Cystic fibrosis: a new outlook. Medicine 56, 129.

34. Kollberg H. 1980. Cystic fibrosis in Sweden: a ten-year sociomedical follow-up. In: Perspectives in cystic fibrosis. Sturgess JM (ed). Toronto: Canadian CF Foundation.
35. Taussig LM, Kattwinkel J, Friedewald WT, di Sant'Agnese PA. 1973. A new prognostic score and clinical evaluation system for cystic fibrosis. Journal of Pediatrics 82, 380.

7. ADOLESCENTS AND FAMILY DISRUPTION THROUGH MARITAL SEPARATION

J.W. VAN SETERS

INTRODUCTION

What knowledge do we have of the impact of parental separation and divorce on children in general? Until the seventies very few studies on children of divorced parents were available. In 1953 Despert's was the first publication (1) offering a psychological understanding of children who had to enter treatment because of their problems with their parents' divorce. More recently Gardner (2), the authoritative child psychotherapist, published his PARENTS' BOOK ABOUT DIVORCE. Dutch publications appeared in 1963 (3) and in the early eighties (4,5). In this period more systematic studies of the non-clinical child of divorce were set up, mainly in the United States. Some studies were of a longitudinal character (6,7). These studies suggest a number of points:

a. Children are greatly affected by the separation of their parents, even when they experience relief because of diminishing tension in the home. It may require many years to adjust to the parental break-up, especially for children whose home-base is going through major changes after the original family unit has been dissolved.
b. Children rework the separation theme along a spiral of different developmental stages. They reorganize their conception of the process according to their growing intellectual and emotional capacities.
c. Divorce-associated experiences may be reactivated when children are confronted with new long-term partners of their parents. They may fear a repetition and, in fact, it not infrequently happens that they are again left by these

partners, whom they may have come to consider as new parents.

d. The period around their own leaving home may also be a delicate one in which divorce-related feelings are revived.

e. Children of divorce often report feeling oversensitive to the unavoidable unpredictabilities of their early intimate relationships with peers.

Current empirical investigations focus on the appraisal of age and gender specific reactions to divorce and subsequent absence of the father (8). Other researchers try to reach a deeper understanding of the implications of the parental break-up for the development and personality formation of the child (see in 9,10). These studies are theoretically directed by the conception that the early bonds between the parent and the child constitute the core of the child's personality. Accordingly, impairment of these bonds should have an impact on the child's personality. In these types of projects, long-term adjustment to divorce is correlated with specific factors in the child and the parent. In particular, parental involvement with their children during the several stages of the separation process has been related to measures of children's developmental progress, their self-esteem, their self-concept and the like. These studies usually concern small non-representative samples of participants and very few have comparison groups. Although the findings are not always corroborated, one is led to conclude that in their short-term adjustment to divorce, children need clear manifestations of sustained caring, preferably by each parent, in order to protect or restore their normal functioning, to maintain normal developmental progress, and to safeguard basically good feelings about themselves. As to their long-term adjustment: few children express very positive feelings about the divorce, with the exception of children who were separated from mentally disturbed parents (6,7). It has been found that children rate the divorce as painful and difficult, and maintain strong loyalty to the pre-divorce family structure, even though their understanding of their parents' problems continues to develop. Understanding interpersonal relationships, and the feeling of having personal control of the consequences of the divorce, are found to be predictive of children's positive adjustment to divorce, independently of age (6,7,8).

More empirical data are needed concerning children's long-term adjustment to divorce. They would be of major importance to divorcing parents and to the helping professions, and might be expected to contribute to defining preventive measures and guidelines for lawyers who handle divorce cases and who sometimes have to decide on the issues of custody and visits.

ADOLESCENTS AND FAMILY BREAK-UP

Assumptions and findings

The general findings referred to above centre around children in divorce situations, but how far do they also apply to adolescents? Supposedly, these have somewhat outgrown their need of close belonging to their parents and are less dependent on their care and support. Consequently, one might expect them to be less affected by the adversities of the family disintegration and to experience less stress. On the other hand, adolescents cannot be expected to take divorce lightly. The prevailing sentiment in our culture rates separation through death or divorce as a major life-stress (11,12). Yeaworth et al. (13) find that adolescents also rate events related to death and separation as the most stressful.

Insights concerning the actual experiences of adolescents are to be found mainly in collected case-studies. Those of Tessman (14) were based on adolescents in treatment for loss of their parent(s), while Troyer (15) collected the stories of hundreds of children of divorce, among whom were several adolescents. These studies illustrate the deep feelings of adolescents who seem in no way less upset by their parents' separation than younger children, although they have more mature coping abilities available to deal with their predicament. They may, however, also be more burdened by divorce-related problems than younger children, as we shall see.

Adolescents' responses

One can roughly distinguish three groups of responses.

a. The responses of those, who like anyone else, old or young, enduring loss, have to accept the hard facts. They have to mourn and their development may come to a temporary stand-still.
b. Regressive behaviour may be the temporary or long lasting result for those adolescents whose development clashes with the unforeseen alterations in the expected life-pattern.
c. Accelerated development may occur in adolescents who either feel relieved from familial tension, or decide that the parental divorce sets them free to find their own way.

Adolescents' distress

Like younger children and like most divorcing parents, adolescents grieve when the hope that things might turn out for the best has to be given up and the togetherness of the family is lost. They share the most universal immediate response to divorce in a culture in which the image of the ideal family is still firmly incorporated. The following remarks of adolescents may illustrate this.

> Ruud (aged 15) had felt for years that separation would be the only solution to his parents' problems, but when they finally split up, he realized 'Now our family has completely gone to pieces. We will never be together again as a whole family. We no longer belong together'.
>
> Lisa (aged 14) lived at boarding-school when her parents parted. Although her father had been away from

home most of the time, Lisa felt 'as though the world had collapsed'. She felt that she could no longer say 'I am going home'.

Many adolescents need energy and time to adjust to their changed perception of the parental home and the separateness of their parents. They may be overwhelmed by their unexpected emotions. Some have a hard time facing up to the social position of a youngster of divorce. Withdrawal and loss of concentration score highest among adolescents' self-reported responses. These 'here and now' responses are not to be considered specific for adolescents. More characteristic may be the tendency to avoid the full emotional impact of the shock by those who tell themselves they are too mature to be shocked. This conviction may be responsible for the persistent signs of anger and depression in this age group (6). I will now turn to more specific conditions in the adolescents' separation predicament.

Family break-up may present specific confusion and/or specific challenges to adolescents

'Normal' development

It is worth briefly reviewing the adolescent's developmental tasks, and the model of so called 'normal' development of adolescents in stable homes. The adolescent's developmental tasks concern:

- becoming independent of the parents, materially and emotionally;
- acquiring a sense of integrity and an individual set of values in order to become a responsible member of society in a new historical period;
- becoming able to feel safe and confident in partner-like relationships.

How does the stable home support the adolescent's development? The classical model of adolescent development involves a gradual emancipation in a back and forth movement. The stable home provides a familiar background for youngsters who, in the process of disengaging, alternate between fighting parental control and comfortably submitting to protective measures of parents who still know better. While they experiment with adult actions, adolescents trust that their parents keep an eye on them and will come to their rescue if something goes wrong. Parents are the closest representatives of the older generation. Their standards of life and conduct are the first to be tested and challenged when their youngsters start constructing a new identity and new convictions. Will the new generation stick to, remodel or reject the old family frame of reference? The role parents play in the establishment of their younsters' intimate relationships may be obscure. However, the confidence they have in their children and the confidence they feel in their own marriage, will be assets in their children's behaviour towards prospective partners.

'Normal' development in a disrupted family?

How can the divorcing family be expected to provide the stable and flexible base which adolescents are supposed to need? How well can adolescents accomplish the task of gradually leaving their parents if these are no longer at home to be left? How can youngsters alternate between fighting parental control and trusting their parents' wisdom, if these have become confused themselves, or have adopted unfamiliar behaviours? Where is the old familiar frame of reference which should be questioned by youngsters who come of age, when divorced parents change their identity more rapidly than their adolescents do? Parents may develop new life-styles and form new opinions. Formerly unassailable values are remodelled or overthrown before the new generation gets a chance to evaluate them. And when problems between parents are considered insoluble, how can youngsters learn from this example how to handle their own interpersonal conflicts constructively?

Family disruption may interfere with normal development

Adolescents often mention their anxieties when they lose trusted parental control and the familiar family routines. Some refrain from new activities. Others start acting out indiscriminately, pretending they do not care any more. The loss of parental reliability presents particular hazards to very young adolescents, who are already experiencing increased stress prior to, or immediately after, the change to secondary school. They may suffer a double loss. In their bewilderment they may cling to behaviour that reminds them of the time when both parents were present to guide them through critical periods. Teachers consider children who are confronted with divorce while they are not yet rooted in the new school system as the most vulnerable group of teenagers of divorce.

> Mieke was in her first year of secondary school when her parents parted. Her father moved to a place of his own. Although she claimed to feel happy for him, she was extremely disappointed when he soon got 'another girlfriend'. On the surface she was interested in her mother's jazzy new life and very fond of her father. But she acted revengefully by creating one school failure after another in spite of her more than average intelligence. She got herself thrown out of four successive schools and kept both her parents busy looking for a new place for her. She ended up in an expensive special school as the last resort. At age 16 she feels she is misplaced, but she realizes that she has no choice, since running away from home several times did not work out well, either.

In adolescents, <u>regressive</u> or <u>confused behaviour</u>, <u>inhibition</u> or <u>depression</u>, in reaction to loss of parental attention or control during or after divorce may occur, and this may be of a rather persistent character. Wallerstein and Kelley (6) suggest that adolescents who have suffered previous losses or severe disappointments may be especially vulnerable.

Family disruption may speed up developmental processes

Although confusion and sadness seem general separation experiences, the more militant adolescents may stand up for themselves and use their growing independence constructively. They may disengage from their parents' problems as a strategic withdrawal, thus safeguarding the continuity of their own development.

> Dick (aged 16) notified the judge that he was not intending to give his opinion as to which parent should have custody. Instead, he proposed to live away from his parents until these had decided the issue. In the end, he did not return home and took care of himself most of the time.

Whether this is genuine or pseudo-independence, the recognition of the right to keep aloof from the parents' insecurities may contribute to the adolescent's feeling that he is an autonomous person, capable of defending his own interests. Disengagement may be a rational decision to control the emotional upheaval caused by the breakdown of the parents' familiar behaviour.

> Peter (aged 16) froze into silence for years to come after his statement that he did not want to discuss divorce matters: 'It would interfere with my concentration. I want to finish school and leave home as soon as possible. Meanwhile I stick to my material belongings; then I know what I am up to'.

Most adolescents do not manage to withdraw immediately. They may be drawn to take the part of one parent, or be immersed in their own disappointment for a period of time. But we see the stronger personalities almost overconsciously take the road to a firm individuation and autonomy.

> Judith chose to stay with her deserted mother when she was 14. She was disgusted with her father and felt her mother needed her. She listened to her endlessly and tried to comfort her. But sensing little change or improvement in her mother's feelings, she judged that she was not a very competent helper and that she had better be less involved and do her own thing.

Adolescents who have been forced to take important decisions on their own without, or with very little, support of their preoccupied parents, may develop a self-reliance which make them feel 'older'. They compare themselves favourably with 'helpless' children of intact homes 'who can't prepare their own food' or 'whose decisions are taken for them by their parents'. Studies are as yet lacking concerning whether adolescents of divorce on the average do show a comparatively stronger self-reliance than adolescents of intact homes. However, one cannot conclude that 'strong' adolescents of divorce will live through the break-up untouched. They may mellow and show more empathy towards their parents later, or they may live in a delicate balance. Some have to realize, in years to come, that they have built up defences that have to be taken down again.

> Mieke (aged 16) did not talk about her parents' separation to anyone for about three years. She was very depressed in that period. Now she says: 'One must talk about one's feelings. Otherwise one might crack-up later, may be when one becomes a mother, or when one is forty or so'.

Some youngsters are sadly aware of their early maturity; they may have gained but they also lacked a care-free teen-age.

So far we can conclude that family break-up may complicate the normal developmental processes and threatens to derail them. On the other hand, the divorce experience may help adolescents to accomplish their task of becoming independent of their parents at a relatively early age. Sometimes one can speak of a developmental spurt following the parental separation.

ADDITIONAL PROBLEMS

I now want to reflect upon some additional problems that may arise for adolescents in the divorce or post-divorce period.

Overburden

Although they probably tend to hide post-divorce family problems, one will find many adolescents overburdened by emotional or material tasks. They may get involved in a complicated relationship with the parent they live with. Parents have fewer reservations towards their near-adult youngsters than towards their younger children. They may turn to them in their distress, confusion and loneliness. They may invite or seduce them to take 'the empty seat' of the parent who is gone. Issues of allegiance and loyalty may create profound conflicts for adolescents who have become their parents' confidantes. Particularly confusing are those parents who send 'double messages': who ask support on the one hand and exercise their old authority on the other hand; or who give up responsibility for their youngster, or demand he or she acts independently, and yet baby him or her.

A complex problem arises for the child who has become very close and supportive of a parent who later meets a new partner. Wallerstein and Kelley (6) consider the loss of this exclusive relationship with a single parent the most grievous one of the whole divorce experience. But a child may also harden in this sort of experiences.

> Tom (aged 15) reports amusedly 'My mother has boyfriends off and on. When she has no one I sleep with her in her bedroom. And when a new friend turns

> up, I move out for a while. I don't mind. I like our way of life'.

The stress of overburden will often show up in school problems. Several adolescent boys told me that they had to seek help because they could not get their home-work done properly. They were -each in different ways- overburdened by a combination of household and emotionally supportive tasks, while the custodial parent was sick, or disabled. When children or adolescents are living with a single parent who is working full-time, one should always be aware of the possibility that the child carries a share of domestic responsibility beyond his or her capabilities.

Disturbing parental sexuality

The separation period may be a sexually confusing and provoking one. Parents may all of a sudden, appear to their children as sexual persons. Not infrequently parents confide their new sexual endeavours to their shocked adolescent youngsters as though they had become peers, thus dangerously approaching, or crossing, the invisible sex or incest barriers.

> During a group therapeutic session a boy of 17 expressed his agony at seeing his divorced father flamboyantly charming not only mature women, but also the boy's girl-friends. The boy felt very embarrassed to have his father as a competitor. He was also disgusted to notice that even the relationship between his father and sister had become rather flirtatious. Several other teen-age boys in the group confided that they felt a same discomfort, watching their divorced fathers' goings-on.

Thus, open or inferred sexual feelings of the parents which are not safely confined to wedlock, may become disturbing to their adolescents. Sexual excitement or bewilderment is produced and may be hard to channel.

> Anne, who 'lost' her father at 11 to a neighbour, fervently started to look for a substitute father under the guise of baby sitting. At 13 she met a man, 20 years older, with whom she started a full-grown sexual relationship, which she, at age 16, still hides from her family.

Such examples are not uncommon.

Provocation of physical aggression

The same may apply to aggression. Not infrequently parents engage in physical fighting during marital disturbance. Even young children may feel responsible and try to prevent outbursts of aggression, for instance remaining present while their divorcing parents are together. Although the generational aggression barrier in our culture is generally very strong, older children and certainly adolescents, experiencing a new feeling of growing physical strength, may be provoked to participate in a fight.

> Jan was 5 when his parents separated. Around puberty he became more and more depressed about divorce-induced questions. He felt extremely insecure as to which parent had been 'right' or not and whom he wanted to live with. At age 16, and by now physically mature, he seized an opportunity to blow off his feelings of stress. When his father hit his mother he did not refrain from using force against his father, in order to 'defend' his mother and to 'restore his sense of honour'. As a result his depression miraculously disappeared.
>
> Anne, at the age of 11 a sturdy girl, felt that she

> had every right to attack the woman who took her father away from her. She hates her father for coming in between and cannot understand why he did not respect the physical expression of her despair.

Rather alarming are police reports (Children's Police Utrecht) stating that a growing number of adolescent boys, living in the custody of their mothers, threaten their mothers, or use open violence against them.

Most divorce situations contain some sort of violence, mental or physical, open or hidden. Children witness or sense this and are affected by it. Many have their own reasons to be angry. Some of them will pick up the example offered by parents who let their divorce fights escalate. Aggressive behaviour may be the only outlet for the resulting stress. For other adolescents, controlling their aggressive impulses may require a great deal of effort.

Feelings of responsibility

In the long run, adolescents may become subject to ambivalence between feelings of responsibility and of irritation. They may have deliberately chosen to stay with a deserted parent. If this parent becomes very dependent and remains single, it will be difficult for the adolescent to decide to leave home, even if she or he is ready for independence. Leaving home may thus be delayed considerably. When an adolescent becomes serious about working away from the home-town or setting up his or her own household, it may be a great relief to see a single parent engage in new activities or a new relationship.

> Ruud took care of his alcoholic mother for four years, until he was 19. He felt 'thwarted in his wish to start his own life'. He knew that he more or less covered his problem by flunking his final exams a few times. Finally he was rescued by the reconciliation of

his parents.

ADOLESCENTS OF LONG-STANDING DIVORCE

What is characteristic of adolescents who as children lived through a family break-up is that they seem to remain keenly aware of divorce-linked processes in the family and in themselves, as we have already seen in some of the examples. Although the divorce usually comes to be accepted as an unalterable permanency, several consequences require undiminished checking and balancing. In particular, the complexities of the separate relationships with the parents may demand constant strategic alertness.

Hyper-loyalty to both parents

The phenomenon of children's unwavering, scrupulous loyalty to both parents is noted with perplexity by all investigators in divorce matters. In order to understand this, I will undertake a rather speculative trip. As already indicated, whether their family divorces or not, children feel in their earliest days that they are safe and all is well, when they are loved by their parents, or parent-substitutes. The striving to be loved motivates much of the child's first activities and is thought to establish the root of awareness of the self. The self, a psychological construct, may be seen as composed of effects and reverberations of previous interactions with others and the external world. It is understandable that a child does not want to have this 'composition' divided because of his parents' decision to part. By remaining loyal to both parents a child tries to conserve the integrity of her or his self. After a separation however, one parent usually has to be given up as a daily companion. Often, the relationship then deteriorates to a certain degree. In the adolescent period we can see striking endeavours to revive faded feelings of loyalty. Sometimes, adolescents are willing to bridge deep gaps of hurt feelings. I often sense a wish to find two valued persons as parents, and cannot avoid thinking that finding this would help the feelings of adolescents as whole persons with a respectable background, in short: with a respectable identity.

> Anne (referred to earlier) says at 16: 'I have not seen my father for five years. I hated him and I am still a little scared. But I will soon try to get in touch with him. I need to hear his side of the story. Children need to hear the opinion of both of their parents. Maybe if I could understand my father now, I could feel better about myself'.

Accompanying the wish to know and understand both parents, there is a tendency to attribute equal value to each of them and achieve a kind of symmetry and inner balance. Perhaps the overt behaviour is to be seen as hyper-loyalty to both parents.

De-emotionalizing the parent(s)

Parents who do not live up to certain standards keep threatening their children's feelings about themselves, and parents whose character or life-style troubles their children may therefore interfere with their development. Their relatively mature social-cognitive abilities enable adolescents to de-emotionalize these parents if necessary. Adolescents of divorce are probably less hindered by the invisible boundaries that keep family members together, than adolescents of intact homes. They have survived when they saw these boundaries break before, and if it serves their own purposes they may seem rather precocious in neutralizing their relationship with a parent. They show a remarkable sophistication in crystallizing their parents into psychological portraits, who have to be coped with rationally, according to the nature of the 'portraits'.

Steve (aged 17): 'I do appreciate my mother. She is enterprising and has many friends. But I run into disagreements with her all the time. They are progressive and I want stability in the community. That's why I decided some time ago to live with my father, who is rigid and cannot change. But I need his steadiness, while I prepare for my finals'.

Michael moved to his father's house at 13. He felt his mother was babying him, because she could not give up mothering in spite of her attempt to become a career-woman. When, age 14, he had finished school in his father's neighbourhood and did not find any school there good enough for the education he wanted, he asked his parents permission to live with another family near a better school. His father, he reasoned, was giving him attention only at the weekends anyway, so they might as well live apart.

Mature and strikingly conscious attempts to establish a personal equilibrium and find the best opportunities for further development amidst often quite complicated family relationships seem to me the most striking characteristics of adolescents of long-standing divorces.

GETTING HELP

Of course, not every adolescent of divorce resolves his or her problems alone. If they feel in difficulties they may at first turn to friends who are in the same predicament. It is understandable that divorce problems are hard to communicate and are often kept secret for considerable lengths of time. Intact families are popular as places in which to relax for some adolescents. School counsellors or mental health physicians may be asked to help with school problems which serve as a good alibi. Sensitive police officers may detect the quest for help in the acting out of some bewildered adolescents who are unable to handle their broken home situations. Currently, services are being developed to assist children, and their separated parents, in their adjustment to the implications of the new life-situation. A striking proportion of adolescents' remarks refer to their belief that only someone who has gone through the same experience is to be trusted, or can be of any help. It is as though children of divorce belong to a slightly different species.

SUMMARY

As we have seen the toppling of the family structure presents specific hazards to the adolescent. The absence of a stable family may complicate the developmental processes. Moreover, adolescents are often compelled to participate in the consequences of the parental separation. In another way the transformed family may evoke new skills, and thus provide a social-learning opportunity. When used constructively, a divorce experience seems to enhance the capacity to assess human relationships realistically and to act accordingly.

The quotations are from interviews with adolescents, who participated in a pilot study of non-clinical children of divorce. The study takes place at the University of Utrecht (Vakgroep Sociale Pedagogie) and is subsidized by the Nederlands Kinderpostzegelfonds. Further insights are derived from interviews and written questionnaires filled out by adolescents on behalf of a study for Jeugd en Samenleving (16).

REFERENCES

1. Despert L. 1953. Children of divorce. New York: Doubleday.
2. Gardner RA. 1977. Parents' book about divorce. New York: Doubleday.
3. Fournier EP. 1963. Kinderen van gescheiden ouders. Deventer: Van Loghum Slaterus.
4. van Seters W. 1980. Kind, gezin en echtscheiding. Deventer: Van Loghum Slaterus.
5. Lichtenbelt R. 1981. Kind van gescheiden ouders. Rotterdam: Donker.
6. Wallerstein JS, Kelley JB. 1980. Surviving the break-up. New York: Basic Books.
7. Kurdek LA, Blisk D, Siesky AE. 1981. Correlates of children's long-term adjustment to their parents' divorce. Developmental Psychology 5, pp. 565-579.
8. Hetherington EM. 1979. Divorce, a child's perspective. American Psychologist 37, pp. 34-55.
9. Journal of divorce.
10. Journal of youth and adolescence.
11. Dohrenwend BS, Dohrenwend BP. (1974). Stressful life events. New York: Wiley.
12. Holmes TH, Rahe RH. 1967. The social readjustment scale. Journal of Psychosomatic Research 11, pp. 213-218.
13. Yeaworth RC, York J, Hussey MA, Ingle ME, Goodwyn T. 1980. The development of an adolescent life change event scale. Adolescence 15, pp. 91-97.
14. Tessman L. 1978. Children of parting parents. New York: John Aronson.
15. Troyer W. 1979. Divorced kids. 1979. Toronto: Clarke, Irwin and Co.
16. Special Issues on Children and Divorce: Jeugd en Samenleving 1979, volume 3/4; 1981, volume 9.

8. EROTIC OVERTURES AND SEXUAL CONTACTS; COMPETENCE, RULES, ATTITUDES AND PROBLEMS

Cornelius J. Straver

SOCIO-EROTIC OVERTURES

Sexuality of adolescents manifests itself to a large degree as a tendency towards contact with a special boy or girl, or with boys or girls in general. Sexuality resides in the admiration for, and in the attraction to, other people. This admiration or attraction materializes in daydreams and fantasies, and stimulates only gradually and slowly the first halting steps to gain the attention and positive attitude of the object. After a period in which interest for the other sex is shown in a more general way through demonstrative behavior towards them in peer groups, personal attempts at an overture are gradually undertaken. The beginning of this process occurs somewhere between the ages of twelve and fourteen, but overture actions and the problems connected with them remain vivid during the whole period of middle and late adolescence and even in adulthood.

In my study on socio-erotic overtures (1) I described these in the framework of an action theory, and distinguished eight steps in the building-up of a socio-erotic overture; i.e. fantasizing, making a plan of action, activating the rules, preparing oneself mentally, initiating and maintaining the actual contact, acting symbolically, negotiating on each other's intentions, and establishing the result.

If one desires to approach someone else one often starts with a global vision of an attractive situation. 'In my fantasy I see myself in contact with the other person, i.e. talking together, doing nice things together, making love etc.'. But reaching such a situation demands a restructuring of the fantasy into a viable plan or design for action, i.e. a number of steps to be taken. This could be a rather vague idea or a more detailed scenario: 'first do this, and then I could do this, etc.'.

A plan includes strategies, which are necessary because one does not know if the other sees oneself in the same way as one sees the other. Plans and strategies include rules: not only or even primarily what is socially acceptable, but especially rules as 'rules of the art'. In fact one uses some, mostly implicit, theories of action: 'If I do this and he/she reacts in such a way it will mean ....' etc. Socially approved schemes of actions will be involved in the rules and action hypotheses. As we will see later, such socially approved action schemes often prove to be dysfunctional regarding the wishes and competencies of young people.

Even when one knows how to behave, having acquired 'the rules of the game', it often happens that courage is lacking. One has to accept and overcome the gulf which exists, by definition, before an overture to a stranger is made. There is the risk of a rebuff and even the ridicule of others. Thus, making an overture presupposes positive self-esteem, as well as the competency to develop an overview of the situation and assess one's chances of success.

Then, at a given moment the first step must be taken. This requires a repertoire of behavior, acquired by watching others and by one's own inventiveness. In order to initiate contact and maintain it for some time, behavioral steps appropriate to the demands of the particular situation must be taken. Maintaining the contact is a condition for the subsequent steps to occur.

In maintaining contact, behavior with symbolic significance is likely to be important. One wants to arouse in the other the emotion which was present in the earlier fantasy. Arousing emotions doesn't happen by rational discussions, but by small expressions of warmth and positive feeling in the tone of speech, eye-contact, and in friendly remarks etc. One could say for instance 'what a nice thing to say', with the connotation of 'what a nice boy you are'. By showing admiration or other positive feelings one hopes to create a warm and positive atmosphere in which the other starts to respond in the same vein, thus initiating a chain reaction.

If attempts so far have been successful, it now becomes important to discover if the object of one's affections has reciprocal intentions. This is likely to involve interpreting small hints coming from the other and, if these are not clear enough, to send further implicit messages to the other concerning the initiatior's intentions, with the aim of clarifying those of the 'object'. In such situations the assumed intentions of the other can easily be misinterpreted, at least in part, and this can lead to a real but subdued struggle for clarifications and agreement. At a given moment the intentions may become clear enough to allow for a more definitive step: telling each other that they want to prolong the contact or to finish it. If both parties want to prolong it, they will usually make an appointment to meet again.

It might be asked if this description of the overture as an action process is only valid for boys, as they are generally supposed to take the initiative. However, the same scheme of steps applies to anyone who takes an active part in an overture. As we will see later, a rather large number of boys are reluctant to assume this role, whereas a larger number of girls is much more active in making overtures than the social stereotype would imply. Moreover, though girls often wish to be more active than social rules seem to allow, they sometimes may not do so out of uncertainty about the boy's feelings. However, even if they restrain themselves and stick to the socially approved rules, girls show several kinds of active behavior, such as moving near to the boy and staying in his vicinity; sending signals by eye movement and body position; reacting to any step taken by the boy in a way which will maintain the contact; acting in a way that conveys symbolic meaning and negotiating further, etc. The girl, too, needs to know the rules of the game and to apply them, whether she follows more traditional patterns (being passive), or more modern ones (going up to a boy and starting a chat). In this context it is significant that boys and girls find it equally difficult to make contact, as we will shortly see.

In our research (2; for additional details see Appendix to this chapter), we find a rather large number of difficulties in making overtures experienced by both boys and girls:

a. Thirty-five per cent of the boys and 40% of the girls find it sometimes or often difficult to make contact with members of their own sex, while 50% of the boys and 44% of the girls experience difficulties in making contact with members of the opposite sex. On the individual level, overtures towards the opposite sex are significantly more often experienced as difficult. However, there is a strong correlation (.61) between problems in the two kinds of overture situation. Such problems may be due to many boys and girls not learning the 'grammar' of social interactions at a younger age.
b. Many young people feel themselves insecure in new contacts. Thus, in this situation, 57% of the boys and 65% of the girls find it sometimes or often difficult to find something to say to a member of the opposite sex.
c. Many boys and girls think that knowing how to make an overture is an inborn quality. Some testify that previously they didn't know how but that they have since learned a lot. In general, both boys and girls realize that an overture has to be 'made', but they do not believe that how to make it can be learned.
d. Boys and girls often behave awkwardly towards an uncertain partner. They may then try to help the other. Boys turn out to be considerably less successful in this than girls. A number of girls however, fend off insecure boys: they want a 'man'.
e. Boys and girls are heavily dependent on their circle of friends to come in contact with new girls or boys. Without

such a circle most youngsters would not have new contacts.

f. The procedures used by boys and girls to make contact are predominantly weak. Fifteen per cent of the boys and 16% of the girls do not know what to do or how to do it. A third of the boys and nearly 40% of the girls behave according to the traditional social scenario: the boy actively approaches the girl, while the girl looks attentive and waits until the boy approaches her. The weak-active form of overture (starting a chat when the opportunity is offered) however, is predominant. We find that it occurs with 40% of the boys and 37% of the girls. Clearly, girls are more active than the social stereotype would allow; boys less active than their social role prescribes.

g. The last mentioned point is confirmed by the stated attitudes of boys and girls: 53% of the boys prefer to await some demonstration of interest in them from the girls, while 46% of the girls admire other girls who actively make overtures to boys.

h. Consistent with these attitudes, 75% of the boys find it acceptable for a girl to come up to them and start a chat, and even more than 50% accept a girl asking them for a dance. Most girls (two thirds) also accept going up to a boy to start a chat. Asking him for a dance, however, is considered unacceptable by most of the girls. Interestingly enough, boys and girls also largely approve of the traditional scenario in which the girl waits and the boy approaches. This double standard, or at least strong ambivalence, means that new scenarios are not clear for the youngsters. They aspire to these but often cannot reach them. This situation is particularly awkward for girls. They do not know what kind of norms the boy they wish to approach will have before the initial contact is made, so they often protect themselves by playing it safe, i.e. waiting until the boy starts the overture. Thus, there is a double misunderstanding between boys and girls regarding the norms for socio-erotic overtures. Firstly, girls do not know that boys are ready to accept active steps from them in overtures, and boys do not know that girls want to behave actively. Secondly, as a result of such ignorance, neither sex tends to behave according to its wishes, thereby confirming the traditional scenarios which many do not want.

In this context it is important to know that we found two different subcultures among youngsters: on the one hand the subculture in which the traditional scenarios predominate; on the other, the subculture of informal friendship-like forms of overture scenarios. The first is more often found in social circles and meeting places of young working-class people; the second in circles and meeting places of young people pursuing higher education. However, the kind of scenario occurring also depends on the type of meeting place. Informal types of overtures are commoner in schools, clubs etc., whereas more traditional scenarios prevail at discos, beaches etc. In general we find that the more impersonal a social situation is, the more young people will lean on traditional scenarios (and the more difficulties youngsters will experience).

Friends, and peers in general, play a very important role in finding scenarios for overtures with the appropriate rules and procedures. Six kinds of contributions by friends and peers may be mentioned here. Firstly, peers stimulate each other's attention to the opposite sex by dramatizing the sex differences (by demonstrative behavior in groups towards the opposite sex, by stories about conquests etc.). The big 'social Gestalts' of love and relationships are made accessible by fractionating them into small steps. Secondly, peers offer a stepwise developmental scale: having a girl- or boy-friend seems already a big leap forward for the youngest group, having some sexual contact (heavy petting) seems a next step for the group which already has some contacts, and so on. Thirdly, peers demonstrate to each other the different basic structures of relating to the opposite sex (conquest versus informal friendship-like contact). Fourthly, peers show different kinds of behavior in making contact and in maintaining contacts, thereby provoking each other with procedures and rules. Fifthly, friends often help to arrange opportunities for making contact. Sixthly, friends provide opportunities for feedback by talking with each other about their personal experiences as in endeavours to make contact, and about the insecurities they have experienced.

In contrast to this role of peers and friends, our research shows that parents contribute little to the establishment of social and erotic contacts (3).

In concluding this section mention should be made of the difficult position of youngsters with 'deviant' desires, such as homosexual feelings. If they already have some awareness of such feelings, and this mostly starts some time during adolescence (4,5), they feel like outsiders in the typical group processes of peers and friends. Often they find themselves in an ambivalent position, trying to play heterosexual roles and repressing their feelings. In fact they are missing an appropriate context in which they could explore their feelings and go through a number of steps comparable to those of their heterosexual peers. This frequently leads to more or less chaotic processes when they later try to catch up in their retarded social development. They often enter homosexual subcultures in which it is frequently difficult to find real partners (as most of them aspire to) due to the artificial and impersonal atmosphere in many of these subcultural milieus, which are mostly in discos and bars. It is only in societies which are tolerant and accepting enough to allow people to 'come out' at an earlier age, that more natural milieus for making contacts and finding partners could develop.

EXPLORATION OF PHYSICAL CONTACTS

The exploration of physical contacts and, connected with it, the exploration of relational perspectives, is a process which evolves in a number of stages from puberty to late adolescence. These stages can be discovered by careful study of the valuable collection of sexual biographies edited by Ribal (6). These stages are: anticipation, gradual and stepwise development, barriers and decisions, the discovery of the relational perspective, the appropriation of relational insight, the awareness of a growing competence.

At the beginning of adolescence youngsters discover the symbolic meaning of the other sex in its outward appearance, shape of body, and modes of conduct etc. They are guided in this process by the demonstrative behavior of the peers, by the 'social Gestalts' in our culture, and by their explorations by watching and fantasizing. They start to develop an anticipation of new experiences and future actions, which now seem possible and attractive. Becoming a grown-up man or woman with sexual and relational experiences starts to be a motivating factor. These anticipations work like a motor which starts and keeps the whole development going. From these anticipations youngsters start their fantasizing and attempts at socio-erotic overtures, which are followed by the exploration of physical nearness by hugging, kissing and necking.

The gradual and stepwise development in learning several grades of physical intimacy is documented by many other inquiries as well as by the biographies. In their study of young German workers, Schmidt and Sigusch (7) describe how the development from first kiss until first coitus in general takes a period of three years, starting at the age of 15-16. Later studies by the same authors as well as by ourselves (8) show that the process now starts earlier (at the age of 12-14), but nevertheless takes a number of years. In the biographies it becomes clear that children's previous sex play does not precipitate the process. At the onset of puberty and adolescence a completely new process begins. Youngsters disparage their childhood experiences and clearly have the feeling that they are now for the first time starting to learn about overtures, first steps towards physical contacts and so on.

The third stage concerns itself with barriers and decisions. Several researchers have reported on the often dissatisfying experience of the first coitus. Nevertheless all youngsters continue to have further coital experiences. This can only be explained by the above-mentioned anticipation of becoming an adult. Each grade of physical contact (necking, petting, petting to climax, coitus) is some kind of initiation into a new field of experiences. Dissatisfying experiences can stop the process for a while, but after some time youngsters usually make the decision to try again and go further. This is clearly demonstrated in the biographies and also in other research. In Kirkendall's research (9) on the decisions of youngsters for not having coitus, it was discovered that such decisions came not only from girls, but very often from boys who felt they were not sufficiently emotionally developed to undertake such a step. Kirkendall observed that the sexual development of youngsters cannot be properly understood solely in terms of the number of steps taken, and without taking account of decisions as an important part of the process. In the biographies, several youngsters, especially girls, show how at a certain moment they take the decision to lose their virginity. They consciously enter intimate situations with boys where coitus is inevitable. Boys sometimes postpone such situations because of their feelings of uncertainty or lack of competence.

The discovery of relational perspectives -the fourth stage- is intimately related to sexual experience. Although several authors, such as Erikson, claim that a certain degree of identity formation and relational intimacy should be reached before starting coital activity, in practice the process often occurs the other way around. Youngsters often reach the phase of coital behavior at a rather young age, especially in Scandinavia and other more liberal countries. They later discover the relational perspective through their psychosocial development and through their experiences with physical contacts. In the sexual biographies one notes several youngsters who learn from experience that physical contact, as such, can be exciting but not personally satisfying. They start longing for more interpersonal relationships during the middle of adolescence. This is not surprising if one looks at the research on friendship development. More personal friendships are built up only in the middle period of adolescence. Douvan and Adelson (10) and others have examined this topic.

The fifth stage is the acquisition of relational insight and competence. The discovery of the relational perspective does not imply the acquisition at the same moment of the insight and competence which are necessary to maintain satisfying personal relationships. In their biographies several youngsters show how they discovered the 'rules of the game' only gradually, through special circumstances such as being together during a longer period of time (e.g. on a vacation), through meeting several partners successively and learning through these relationships, and through the discovery of the pleasures connected with an intimate relationship.

The feeling of competence -the sixth step- evolves gradually near the end of adolescence. In their descriptions, youngsters maintain that this feeling occurs after they have gone through various processes in relation to the opposite sex: the overture attempts, the elementary and more complex physical contacts, their partial dissatisfaction with these contacts, and their experiences with several successive partners in gradually more satisfying relationships.

In concluding this section, three kinds of problems youngsters experience in physical contacts merit particular mention: feelings of being overwhelmed, problems with initiating physical intimacies, and problems of functioning during such intimacies.

In our research (8), feelings of being overwhelmed are seen in affirmative answers to questions concerning 'being afraid of sexual impulses', 'finding it difficult to control sexual impulses' etc. With boys there is a correlation with answers that demonstrate a certain preoccupation with sex ('am I sex crazy'), and also correlations with level of physical experience and permissive attitudes (-.26 and -.30) (in both cases there are less strong feelings of being overwhelmed). With girls the same feelings are a component of a more general feeling of discouragement in the initiation of physical contacts. Feelings of these kinds do not correlate with statements of aversion to sexuality which were found in only a very few youngsters (contrary to research with middle class adults (11)). The feelings of being overwhelmed, in the light of other correlations in the data, should be interpreted as feelings of interest and appetite.

Problems with initiating physical intimacies show themselves (in our research) by the answers of both boys and girls to questions about: 'how long should you know each other before starting physical intimacies?', 'how should you behave in petting situations in order to maintain a pleasant contact with your partner?'. Boys, especially, worry about how to behave in such a way as to stimulate a girl's interest in physical intimacies: 'how do I start petting while preventing anxiety on the part of the girl?', 'if I want to start heavy petting do I have to neck and hug first?', 'how do I remain aware of both the emotional and physical content of the situation?'. Girls especially worry about how to steer the boy towards being more aware of her wishes: 'could boys pay more attention to my wishes?', 'is it wrong to show to a boy that I am not too interested in physical contact?'. Girls also show more communication problems: 'I have nobody to talk to about sex'.

As regards functional problems in physical intimacies, boys are more directed towards physical gratification and concerned about uncertainties in the sex act. This is shown in the answers to the following questions: 'do I come too quickly?', 'what do I do if the girl is rather passive?', 'what do I do if the girl does not reach orgasm?'. 'what do girls experience when they reach orgasm?' Girls are more directed towards the steering of the boy in the process: 'how do I show the boy that I am willing to have sex?', 'how do I show him that his penetration causes me pain?', 'how do I get him to do more hugging, necking and petting before we start coitus?', 'what do boys experience when they reach orgasm?'. The worries of boys and girls reach high percentages: two-third to three-quarter of the boys and girls do worry about the above-mentioned topics sometimes or often. There is a correlation between the kind of problems experienced and the stage of physical intimacy which has been reached: problems with initiating physical intimacy are mainly found with youngsters who are petting under the clothes (girls .49, boys .20), while problems with functioning in physical intimacies are mainly experienced by those who have reached the stage of coital behavior (girls .39, boys .46).

THEORETICAL AND PRACTICAL DISCUSSION

The foregoing description of the sexual development of youngsters is not a direct result of the physiological changes during puberty, as is often assumed by psychologists and physicians. Physiological changes have no integrative power and do not lead to the discovery of the relational perspective or of the symbolic meaning of the opposite sex. For this, we have to take as our starting point mental development as described by cognitive psychologists like Jean Piaget and his followers (13,14). He calls attention to a new phase in cognitive development beginning around the age of 11-12 years, and called the formal-operational type of thinking. It means that the youngster starts to progress from the concrete-operational thinking typical of the elementary school period, and that he becomes able to distinguish between what is actually given and what is possible. It is no longer necessary that the given situation be as it is: it could be different. This leads to 'de-centring', the ability to look critically at a situation as though from the outside, and sometimes to criticism for its own sake. Parents and adults in general are seen as not realizing what they could and should do. Parallel with this process the youngster becomes able to idealize, to dream about utopias, but also to discover values. The obverse of this development is that the youngster is forced to evaluate himself: he sees himself through the eyes of others and can be strongly disappointed about his appearance, his conduct, and his life. His own appearance as well as that of others are seen in the light of values and of what they promise. The other person can assume the guise of a promise of some positive and attractive fulfilment. The symbolic perception of the other is born, and with this the symbolic perception of the other sex becomes possible (e.g. 12). In his further development the youngster becomes able to put himself in the position of the other, and he learns that while being with another he will nevertheless (or even more strongly) remain with himself. This double experience of being with the other while experiencing oneself opens for him the discovery of the relational perspective and the exploration of the subtleties of a relationship.

The first section of this paper (on socio-erotic overtures) was not presented in terms of a developmental perspective, but as an application of action theories which came to the fore at the beginning of the seventies (see e.g. 14,15). Action theory means that behavior is studied as it is made ('constructed') by the actor in view of a goal or anticipation. Social reality is studied as it emerges from the actions of a person, mostly in relation to his social or physical environment. The emerging action is followed through the several phases of its construction, as was done with the socio-erotic overtures. We can also recognize something of the context of this action process of socio-erotic overtures (from the data of our research with a representative sample of 1.000 Netherlands youngsters of age 15-21 years). The strong connection between overture problems with the opposite sex and with own sex pointed towards a lack in the learning of the general grammar of social relationships. The practical conclusion from this piece of research is, therefore, that youngsters need to learn to master that grammar at a young age.

Parents and schools could play an important role by helping the child to overcome shyness, to learn to express feelings etc. At the University at Groningen, Dr Sanders of the Institute of Social Psychology has started an experimental program to help youngsters at the beginning of their high school period (age 13-14) to learn several aspects of relating to other people, by using games, role playing and discussions. The intention of this program is not so much to do what 'shyness clinics' are doing, nor is it a training to learn erotic overtures. Using a multiplicity of methods, the youngsters learn to master social relations in a broad area of applications. The supposition is that learning social grammar in general will help tremendously in more specific areas like socio-erotic overtures and physical contacts. These areas are just specific examples of general social contacts. The same grammar with its basic rules should be applicable to the whole field. Special attention is given to the training of assertiveness, thereby helping to acquire or reinforce self-confidence. The program aims at teaching junior high school teachers to apply these techniques in some specific classes and is not a program that could only be implemented by specialists. At the moment we still have to await the outcomes of these experiments.

APPENDIX

THE SAMPLE AND METHOD OF INVESTIGATION

The investigation was commissioned by the Dutch government - or more specifically, by the ministries responsible for youth affairs and for public health. Our aim was to interview a representative sample of Dutch juveniles between the ages of 15 and 21; the total sample was to comprise 1.000 young people and 550 of their fathers or mothers. References made in this report apply primarily to that part of the investigation applying to the young people.

The sample was obtained by randomly selecting young people from population registers in 63 randomly chosen cities, stratified according to region and degree of urbanization. Four per cent of the youths designated to be interviewed proved to be living elsewhere, and 5% had not been encountered at home after three visits. Fifteen per cent of the total sample refused to be interviewed, while 7% of the parents refused permission for the interview. In all, 29% of the sample refused to cooperate in the investigation. Not being at home, or living somewhere else, was more common for young people who worked than for those who were still in school. We therefore have a slight over-representation of youths attending school (7%). The parents of younger girls and boys refused permission relatively more often, while older boys themselves refused relatively more often to be interviewed. It is therefore probable that we have on the one hand too few young people with conservative parents, and on the other hand too few older boys who are sexually experienced. This presumably has little effect upon the average of the answers, since the no-response cases are most likely to have occurred at both extremes. The range of the answers is likely to be slightly too limited as a result. At the end of the written part of the questionnaire, 6% of the boys and 4% of the girls indicated that they had not answered honestly. On the other hand, more than half of the young people said that they had told or written down things which they had kept hidden from everyone until then.

Structured questionnaires were used in the investigation with preponderantly pre-coded answers and several open questions. Most of the interview was carried out orally; written lists were used for five topics (knowledge questions, taking stock of problems, sexual experience). These written questionnaires were filled in by the respondent during the interview, with the interviewer being careful not to look over their shoulder while they did it; the interviewee put the completed form in an envelope, sealed it, and gave it to the interviewer at the end of the interview.

Advanced students in the Social Sciences were used as interviewers; they already had had experience in interviewing, and received supplementary interview training (making use of role-playing, instruction, etc.). Each young person was interviewed by someone of the same sex, and more or less the same age. Only the interviewer and interviewee were present during the interview. On the average the interview lasted two hours.

A limited number of category classifications was developed for handling the material obtained from the small number of open questions by making an initial inventory of the answers. The answers were then doubly coded. The agreement among the coders was in general extremely high. The pre-coded and newly coded questions were then transferred to a code list (sheet) and then fed into the computer by means of a tape. Both cross tabulations and correlations were computed for the material; in addition, a large number of regression analyses were carried out on the material in order to see which independent variables make a contribution to what degree to which dependent variables (behavior, problems, attitudes, knowledge, etc.).

Several weeks later the father and mother of something more than half of the young people were questioned one at a time (percentage of refusals 13%). This took place in the form of an interview with primarily pre-coded, and several open questions. The conversations were carried out by other, older interviewers, who knew nothing about the answers of the young people. These older interviewers also had had extensive interview experience and also received supplementary training and instructions. The material was coded and manipulated in the same way as for the young people. During the analysis the data obtained from young people was coupled with that obtained from the parents.

The investigation was reported in three volumes (2,3,8) in which were treated respectively: a) approach behavior and problems connected with it; b) sex behavior in relationships, problems and attitudes, c) attitudes of parents and how they help young people. This article only deals with parts of volume a and b.

REFERENCES

1. Straver CJ. 1980. Jong zijn en contact zoeken. Deventer: Van Loghum Slaterus.
2. Straver CJ, de Boer J. 1977. Toenaderingsgedrag van jongens en meisjes. Zeist: Nisso.
3. de Boer J. 1979. Behoedzame ontmoediging. Zeist: Nisso.
4. Moerings M. 1970. Homofiele jongeren in relatie tot hun omgeving. Zeist: Nisso.
5. Sanders GJEM. 1977. Het gewone en het bijzondere van de homosexuele leefsituatie. Deventer: Van Loghum Slaterus.
6. Ribal JE. 1973. Learning sex roles; American and Scandinavian contrasts. San Francisco: Canfield.
7. Schmidt G, Sigusch V. 1971. Arbeiter-Sexualitaet. Neuwied: Luchterhand.
8. Straver CJ, de Boer J. 1978. Gevoelige kwesties omtrent sexuele contacten van jongens en meisjes. Zeist: Nisso.
9. Kirkendall LA. 1967. Characteristics of sexual decision making. Journal of Sex Research 3, 201-211.
10. Douvan E, Adelson J. 1966. The adolescent experience. New York: Wiley.
11. Frenken J. 1976. Afkeer van sexualiteit. Deventer: Van Loghum Slaterus.
12. Elkind D. 1968. Cognitive development in adolescence. In: Understanding adolescence. Adams JF (ed). Boston: Allyn & Bacon.
13. Piaget J. 1954. The construction of reality in the child. New York: Basic Books.
14. Piaget J, Inhelder B. 1969. The psychology of the child. New York: Basic Books.
15. Mischel Th. 1969. Human action; conceptual and empirical issues. New York: Academic Press.
16. Harré P, Secord PF. 1972. The explanation of social behavior. Oxford: Blackwell.

9. SEX ROLES AND COPING WITH EMOTIONS

W. EVERAERD

Growing up a male or female is likely to result in coping with disturbances in different ways. In this chapter I will concentrate on these differences, starting from the observation that males are more defensive in comparison to females when they meet threatening situations (1). It is a common experience in assistance situations that males are less prepared to seek help, they refuse help more frequently, and their drop-out in therapy is higher in comparison to females. Yet there is some evidence that during growing up, males experience more threats, especially threats to their emotional well-being. From my experience with adults in the field of sexology, it has become clear that males are more helpless than females as a consequence of sexual dysfunctions, surgical interventions, and problems in relation to their sexual orientation (paraphilias). In many cases these problems seem to represent a severe blow to their male identity, with disastrous consequences. Although these differences may to some extent be explained in terms of sociosexual competence, as is beautifully demonstrated in Straver's chapter (chapter 8 in this volume), specific aspects of male role behavior on an individual psychological level may be an important causal factor. Sex differences in coping with emotional threats can be attributed to two sources. Biologically orientated explanations are in line with Money's concept of male vulnerability (2). Psychological and sociological explanations deal with clarifying how cultural stereotypes of the female and male role and behavior have been learned.

VULNERABILITY

Male vulnerability is documented from many sources (2). It starts with the suggestion that there is a greater loss of male concepti during pregnancy. A high mortality rate in utero results from the malfunction or malformation of many developing male embryos. In economically deprived families there seem to be more girls than boys. Males seem to be more vulnerable to many childhood diseases. They are prone to both learning and emotional disorders. Money (2) reported a larger incidence of psychosexual disorders in males. Female disorders in this area might have been hidden and ignored by societies. However, there are also less clinical reports of female psychosexual disorders.

Reinisch et al. (3) refer to greater difficulties in male, than in female, differentiation. They suggest that three factors may be of particular importance. Firstly, androgen must be present in sufficient amounts and at the appropriate times. In its absence demasculinization or feminization may ensue. Since male development is more complex, there are more opportunities for an error to occur. A second contributing factor is that the Y-chromosome carries less genetic information than the second X-chromosome in the female, so that sex-linked characteristics such as color-blindness, baldness, and hemophilia are more common in males than in females. Reinisch et al. suggest a third contributing factor, namely greater rigidity in rearing male offspring. This might be a consequence of the much more narrow definition of masculinity than femininity in western cultures.

Rigidity in the definition of masculinity and thus in male behavior, may however, be as much adaptive as maladaptive, in that it may facilitate many male achievements. In the face of emotional threats, however, it sometimes becomes a disturbing defense. Dominance, aggression and defensiveness tend to be differentially learned more by boys than girls (4).

SEX ROLES

Schoof-Tams et al. (5) report that sociosexual contacts between boys and girls in the seventies are guided by egalitarian concepts. Nevertheless, equality is limited. There are still traditional role expectations as regards the sharing of duties in marriage and the taking of sexual initiatives. In a recent study of American college students males and females indicated that they both accepted and practised traditional sexual scripts. Men used any available strategy to have sexual intercourse and women used any available strategy to avoid it (6). From an on-going study at our institute it was found that males who are active participants in male liberation were reported to be more egalitarian in sharing initiative and power with their female partners. In most cases this increased equality was a result of females striving for it. Although these men considered their relationships as egalitarian, they still reported that they were more active, and gave more in their sexual interactions, as compared with their female partners. In terms of a stereotyped image of male role behavior, the most likely interpretation of this finding is that even these men were controlling their emotions by defining their sexual relationships in terms of who is doing what, and to whom, instead of concentrating on their feelings.

Masters and Johnson (7) reported these stereotyped role behaviors as being specific to heterosexual interactions as compared with homosexual interactions. Thus it seems to be especially difficult to grow up as a heterosexual male when we look at how these male cope with (sexual) emotions.

SEX DIFFERENCES IN CHILDHOOD

Most studies on sex differences are concerned with cognitive abilities and motor skills (8). Emotional development has been studied in achievement situations (9). The focus of this research was the differential treatment of boys and girls by their teachers and parents in cases of success and failure. In spite of being better achievers in school situations, girls tend to attribute their failures to lack of ability, while boys attribute them to lack of effort or persistence. Faced with failure, girls seem to become helpless while boys attribute it to controllable factors. However, boys tend to attribute success to their abilities more readily than do girls.

There is some evidence for similar reactions of males and females when they are confronted with other disturbing emotions. In pre-school children there are almost no consistent sex differences in emotional expression (10), although there is a possible slight tendency for boys to be more distressed by novel stimuli. Studies reviewed by Rutter found that more boys appeared frightened by a novel toy monkey that clapped cymbals, whereas girls tended not to be distressed. Significantly more boys than girls were distressed when first attending an experimental playgroup. Boys were found to be more likely to cry than girls as a result of frustration. Young boys seem to have a lower frustration threshold, they are more aggressive and impulsive and they get into quarrels and fights more often than girls. Boys would therefore be more likely to get into conflicts with parents and teachers because of their aggressiveness, and this in turn, would increase the amount of stress they experience.

A further factor creating problems for young boys concerns the more stringent sex role expectations for boys than for girls. At an early age the boy learns that he is expected to be masculine and that he must earn a masculine identity. Young girls are allowed to succeed in traditionally masculine activities, and it is only in adolescence that they are expected to behave in a feminine manner. Not only is the range of appropriate behaviors smaller for boys but they are also more likely to find it difficult to maintain appropriate role behaviors, as they are immersed in a feminine world both at home and in school. In this world both boys and girls may be unconsciously rewarded for feminine behavior. Female nursery school teachers rewarded boys a total of 232 times for sex-preferred behaviors and of these,

199 were feminine behaviors (11, p. 28). In comparison girls were reinforced 363 times, with 353 of the reinforcements for feminine behaviors. As appropriate sex role behavior is primarily learned as a consequence of contacts with persons of the same sex, it would appear that boys have much more limited opportunities for such learning.

THE TRANSITION TO ADULTHOOD

During the transition from childhood to adulthood sex differences change markedly. From self-report anxiety scales in later childhood it was found that girls are somewhat more willing than boys to admit that they feel anxious (10).

An interesting explanation for this change is proposed by Gove (11). For young boys the clearest problem is that although their intellectual and physical development is slower than that of girls they are expected to perform as well as girls. It appears that boys experience a greater difference between their ability and the expectations of others than do girls. It should follow that boys experience more stress than girls.

For young boys, as we have seen, sex role behavior is somewhat problematic. However, when they enter the more masculine adolescent world they seem to have acquired a masculine identity and have relatively few problems meeting the sex role expectations. At adolescence girls are suddenly confronted with strong pressures to conform to the feminine role, which is bound to induce some role conflict and anxiety. The adolescent girl's sex role tends to be narrower than that of boys. A very basic assumption in our society is that adolescent and adult females will defer to men and adopt traditional female aspirations and behavior. Yet at the same time women are told that they are the equals of men and have equal opportunities. Thus the female is confronted with the choice of competing with the masculine world at the cost of denying herself as a women, or of responding to the covert message by deferring to men. Further, the feminine role focuses on inter-personal ties with males, depending at the same time on the actions of males. It is very likely that females find this uncertainty and lack of control over their future very frustrating.

Gove (11) reviews much empirical evidence for the differential socialization of boys and girls. His explanation for the transition from young childhood to adolescence may be summarized: when adolescents prepare to move into the adult roles they become aware that males are favored in our society and girls start experiencing the stress associated with their adult sex role. Hence, it would appear that by late adolescence, girls would experience as much stress, and probably more, than boys (11, p. 31). In the development of sexual orientation during the transition from childhood to adolescence, aspects of sex roles have been stressed as underlying the development of sexual preferences. Bell et al. (12) found gender role non-conformity to be a contributing factor in the development of homosexuality. They inferred from their results that this is more salient in males than in females. Males are more often thought to have to prove or earn the designation 'masculine', whereas being 'feminine' for a female is more of an ascribed status which is not questioned unless the girl's behavior invites it. In other words, boys have to actively do things to show that they <u>are</u> masculine, while girls have to actively do things to show that they <u>are not</u> feminine.

Storms (13) speculates that the time of onset of puberty (early or late) and the pattern of social bonding (early = homosocial, late = heterosocial) interact to produce homo- and heterosexual orientation, though he admits that the causal chain cannot be decided from available data. However, in contrast to Bell and his associates (12), Storms found no evidence in his research concerning non-conformity and sex role behavior (13).

SEX ROLES AND ATTITUDES TOWARD PSYCHOLOGICAL HEALTH

Non-conformity to sex roles seems to play an important role in attitudes toward psychological health. Heilbrun (14) reports data on the dissimulation of self-descriptions on masculinity and femininity scales (table 1). Subjects were instructed to appear as psychologically healthy as possible ('fake good') and then to simulate a psychologically unhealthy person ('fake bad'). In the

Table 1. Effect of 'fake good' and 'fake bad' instructions on masculinity and femininity scores (14).

	'Fake good'		'Fake bad'	
	Males	Females	Males	Females
Masculinity scale	56.46	52.68	43.32	51.26
Femininity scale	46.30	46.42	32.82	19.58

'fake good' condition males and females did much the same thing. They described themselves as slightly more masculine and slightly less feminine than average scale norms. This seems to support the assumption that masculine behaviors are more highly esteemed than feminine behaviors. However, in the 'fake bad' condition males dropped their masculinity scale scores while females maintained their masculinity scale scores. A loss of masculinity was an important aspect of the male's concept of psychological adjustment. The most salient effect of the instructions appears in the femininity scale scores. Femininity scale scores were not high under 'fake good' instructions but dropped under 'fake bad' instructions. According to Heilbrun the absence of feminine tendencies is central to the concept of psychological health for both sexes. The marked drop in femininity scale scores in females can lead to a somewhat modified conclusion; in both sexes poor psychological health is seen as involving less conformity with their own sex role.

Heilbrun's findings are to a large extent corroborated in studies on sexual dysfunctions. Males and females with sexual dysfunctions are found to use less adjectives from masculinity and femininity scales when compared with non-dysfunctional males and females. Dysfunctional females seem to be more depressed and have lower self-esteem as compared with non-dysfunctional females. Dysfunctional males tend to maintain their self-esteem by behaving more sex-typically. They appear more masculine or instrumental and less feminine or expressive (15,16).

Kagan (17) said, in describing the basis for sex differences in behavior, that 'the primary covert attributes in sex role standards for men include a pragmatic attitude, sexual prowess and capacity, and the ability to control the expression of strong emotions that signify weakness, especially fear, sorrow and loneliness' (p. 94).

The initial male vulnerability seems to be socialized towards invulnerability. In the face of disturbing emotions they appear as masculine, a helpless defence when confronted with weakness.

REFERENCES

1. Pleck JH. 1981. The myth of masculinity. Cambridge, Massachusetts: MIT Press.
2. Money J. 1977. Determinants of human gender identity/role. In: Handbook of sexology. Money J, Musaph H (eds). Amsterdam: Elsevier, pp. 57-79.
3. Reinisch JM, Gandelman R, Spiegel FS. 1979. Prenatal influences on cognitive abilities: data from experimental animals and human endocrine syndromes. In: Sex related differences in cognitive functioning. Witting MA, Peterson AC (eds). New York: Academic Press, pp. 215-239.
4. Maccoby EE, Jacklin CN. 1974. The psychology of sex differences. Stanford: Stanford University Press.
5. Schoof-Tams K, Schlaegel J, Walczak L. 1976. Differentiation of sexual morality. Between 11 and 16 years. Archives of Sexual Behavior 5, 353-370.
6. LaPlante MN, McCormick N, Brannigan GG. 1980. Living the sexual script: college students' views of influence in sexual encounters. Journal of Sex Research 16, 338-355.
7. Masters W, Johnson V. 1979. Homosexuality in perspective. Boston: Little, Brown and Company.
8. Jacklin CN. 1979. Epilogue. In: Sex related differences in cognitive functioning. Wittig MA, Peterson AC (eds). New York: Academic Press, pp. 357-371.
9. Dweck CS, Goetz TE. 1978. Attributions and learned helplessness. In: New directions in attribution research, vol. 2. Harvey JH, Ickes W, Kidd RF (eds). New York: Wiley, pp. 158-179.
10. Rutter M. 1980. Emotional development. In: Scientific foundations of developmental psychiatry. Rutter M (ed). London: Heinemann, pp. 306-321.
11. Gove WR. 1979. Sex differences in the epidemiology of mental disorder: evidence and explanation. In: Gender and disordered behavior. Gomberg ES, Franks V (eds). New York: Brunner and Mazzel, pp. 23-68.
12. Bell AP, Weinberg MS, Hammersmith SK. 1981. Sexual preference: its development among men and women. Bloomington: Indiana University Press.
13. Storms MD. 1981. A theory of erotic orientation development. Psychological Review 88, 340-353.
14. Heilbrun AB. 1981. Human sex-role behavior. New York: Pergamon.
15. Derogatis LR, Meyer JK. 1979. A psychological profile of the sexual dysfunctions. Archives of Sexual Behavior 8, 201-223.
16. Everaerd W. 1981. Current research in sex therapy. In: Learning theory approaches to psychiatry. Boulougouris J (ed). New York: Wiley, pp. 165-170.
17. Kagan J. 1976. Psychology of sex differences. In: Human sexuality in four perspectives. Beach F (ed). Baltimore: Johns Hopkins University Press, pp. 87-114.

10. OUTPATIENT SOCIAL SKILLS TRAINING FOR YOUTH IN TROUBLE; THEORETICAL BACKGROUND, PRACTICE AND OUTCOME

N.W. Slot and A.A.J. Bartels

INTRODUCTION

In recent years interest in social skills training (SST) has increased. In their review of approximately 150 social skills training experiments Twentyman and Zimering (1) mention the following populations: college students, psychiatric patients, kindergarten-children, alcoholics, mothers of children with behavioral disorders, people with inadequate sexual behaviors, unemployed, and delinquents. Their study, and Bellack and Hersen's reader 'RESEARCH AND PRACTICE IN SOCIAL SKILLS TRAINING' (2) make clear that the various training programs differ strongly from each other.

SST is not just one standard approach and therefore general statements about possible applications or outcome cannot be made. SST emphasizes the acquiring of new skills. Insight into problems, or a high level of verbal functioning, are not necessarily a prerequisite for this form of therapy. This makes it accessible for underprivileged populations.

In this chapter theoretical backgrounds, practice, and outcome-results of an outpatient SST-program are described. The program has been developed at the 'Ambulatorium van het Paedologisch Instituut' in Amsterdam. In chapter 11 in this volume the design, implementation and evaluation of a residential SST are discussed. Both training programs were directed to the specific needs of adolescents with serious problems in their environment, and with maladaptive behavior which brought them to the attention of the juvenile court. We prefer to call them 'youths in trouble', rather than 'juvenile delinquents'. We consider the label 'delinquent' stigmatizing and from a therapist's point of view misleading, since the delinquent behavior often turns out to be just one aspect of serious psychosocial problems.

THEORETICAL BACKGROUND; THE BEHAVIOR DEFICIENCY MODEL

The SST-program was based on the assumption that delinquent as well as non-delinquent behavior is learned. Pavlov's and Thorndike's experiments and the work of Bandura and Kanfer have led to several theories and principles concerned with the learning of behavior. Behavior therapy is based upon these principles and theories. Kanfer (3) makes a distinction between four paradigms, each paradigm consisting of corresponding principles and theories. Three of them will be discussed briefly. The fourth, the classical conditioning paradigm, is less important for the clarification of theoretical backgrounds of SST, and will therefore not be discussed here.

The operant conditioning paradigm

If a specific stimulus elicits a certain behavior which leads to a positive experience, then this behavior is likely to occur in future. Conversely, the behavior will occur less frequently if an unpleasant experience followed. This common sense notion is the basis of the operant conditioning paradigm which emphasizes the mechanism by which the learning of behavior through reward and punishment takes place. Reward is the occurrence of positive events (positive reinforcement) or the absence of aversive events (negative reinforcement). Punishment is the presentation of aversive events or the cessation of positive events. A great amount of empirical research shows that the way in which reinforcements or punishments follow behavior, has a specific impact on the learning of behavior. Continuous reinforcements lead to a high frequency of a particular behavior. Intermittent reinforcement, which means that not every response is followed by reinforcement, results in a high response maintenance. Also the non-existence of behavior can be explained with the aid of operant learning principles. The non-appearance of a certain behavior means that the behavior itself has been extinguished by means of punishing consequences, or that the person has learned escape behavior which excludes the performance of the behavior appropriate to the specific situation, or that the behavior never was reinforced.

For practical therapeutic use the operant paradigm has the following implications:

- In assessing problem behavior the therapist does not only take into account the behavior by itself, but also considers the events preceding the behavior (the stimuli) and the consequences of the behavior.
- The therapist makes an analysis of the pattern by which reinforcements and punishments are established, the so-called functional analysis.
- To produce a change in the problem behavior the therapist tries to change the stimulus, and/or the consequence patterns which maintain the problem behavior.

The model-learning paradigm

This paradigm is associated with the name of Bandura (4). Model-learning theory emphasizes that behavior can be learned through observation. A developing child, for example, acquires new behavior through contacts with different grown-ups and peers, all functioning as models. The child will imitate behavior of such a model, even though it has never been reinforced or punished for practising the behavior. Grown-ups can also learn behavior through observation and imitation of models.

The implications of this paradigm for the therapeutic action are the following:

- Assessing the problem behavior, the therapist takes into account the present and past surroundings of the client. Were there models from whom the client learned his maladaptive behavior, or were models for the desired behavior lacking?

- In order to change the problem behavior the therapist her/himself may decide to act as a model for the client so that the latter learns the desired behavior. This may happen 'in vivo' but also during role-play sessions.
- The therapist may decide to act as a model for nurses, teachers, or family of the client. In this way the therapist can transfer her/his skills to persons who are in frequent contact with the client in her/his natural environment. This procedure is called <u>mediation therapy</u> (5).

The self-regulation paradigm

The name of Kanfer (6) is associated with the self-regulation paradigm. Kanfer emphasizes the way in which people <u>teach themselves behavior</u>. People do this by applying operant learning principles: they reinforce or punish their own behavior. This is done covertly. A certain behavior may be rewarded by thinking: 'good job'. Kanfer differentiates between three stages of self-regulation:

1) self-observation (knowing how one's behavior looks from an observer's viewpoint);
2) self-evaluation (to evaluate personal behavior by means of a standard which is in accordance with the performance of the behavior until now);
3) self-reinforcement (to let a positive or negative consequence follow when the standard has or has not been met).

The implications of the self-regulation paradigm for the therapist are the following.

- Assessing the problem behavior, the therapist determines whether the client is capable of self-observation, and whether the client has realistic standards with regard to her/his own behavior. Especially in the case of youth in trouble these two skills seldom occur. For instance, they do not have the slightest idea how they contribute to the quarrels at home.

- The therapist may change the client's problem behavior by teaching her/him self-regulation techniques. For this purpose self-observation in role-play with the aid of video-taping, self-evaluation by discussing standards for their own behavior, and self-reinforcement, are practised with the client.

DELINQUENT BEHAVIOR AS A BEHAVIOR LACK: THE BEHAVIOR DEFICIENCY MODEL

From a behavioral point of view there are two ways in which problem behavior can be changed:

1) The problem behavior itself is tackled with the aid of response diminishing techniques. In this case the objective will be: reduction or disappearance of the problem behavior, or a change in the client's attitude, and that of those in his immediate environment so that the behavior in question is no longer regarded as a problem.
2) Emphasis is placed on the acquiring of alternative behavior which is incompatible with the maladaptive behavior.

What will determine the choice of these two strategies?

- The seriousness of the problem behavior. Harmful behavior, like self-mutilation, calls for response diminishing procedures.
- The degree to which the client herself/himself regards the behavior as a problem. A client who believes that there is nothing wrong with a certain maladaptive behavior can hardly be expected to participate in a response-elimination procedure.
- If the problem behavior is associated with extreme anxiety it may be undesirable to do something about the behavior directly. In some cases the exposure to stress-provoking stimuli during therapy sessions causes clients to quit therapy.
- The etiology of the problem behavior: response elimination procedures with the aid of punishment for instance, are contra-indicated when the problem behavior has been learnt by avoiding negative consequences (escape behavior). These

techniques may put the client in an extreme stress conflict forcing him/her to 'choose' between two sorts of punishment.

In many therapies both strategies are simultaneously applied: elimination of the problem behavior is combined with the acquisition of new behavior.

However, in our training programs for youth in trouble, we almost always chose to teach new behavior. We explored which behavior the youngsters had not learnt and emphasized the learning of skills which could replace the delinquent behavior. This approach is called the behavior deficiency model (7). We chose this model for several reasons:

1) The literature shows a relationship between deficiencies of social skills and delinquency. Aiken et al. (8) compared delinquent adolescents to their non-delinquent brothers and found that, compared to the latter, they lack social skills. Various other studies (9,10,11) amongst Dutch and Belgian youths suggest that delinquent youths very often have a low self-esteem. This does not automatically warrant the conclusion that low self-esteem implies a lack of social competency. However, summarizing the results of various studies, the connection between social skill deficiencies and delinquency seems strong enough to justify the choice for the deficiency model as a treatment hypothesis. We do not mean to imply, however, that delinquency originates from a deficiency of social skills. Our concern is the choice of a treatment strategy. When youngsters in trouble appear to have few social skills, the unlearning of delinquent behavior is highly undesirable since delinquent behavior often has a function for the youth. They get positive reinforcements like admiration from peers, a thrill and financial rewards. A more profound discussion of the relationship between delinquency and lack of social skills is that by Bartels (12).
2) Delinquent adolescents are seldom aware that they have problems. At the termination of a sentence by the juvenile court they often hold the opinion that their offences, and the problems which went with these, are over and done with. When

they talk about their offences they often maintain that the fault lies with others or in society. High youth unemployment seems, at least partly, to confirm their views on society. Talking about offences and problems often makes them feel very discomfitted and the therapist is easily identified with the punisher. This objection does not hold for the training of alternative behavior in the form of social skills training, especially when the training is made attractive.

3) In 1973, at the start of our study, evidence of the effectiveness of a semi-residential SST-program for youth in trouble had been established. For further reading we refer to the Achievement Place program (7,13).

OUTPATIENT SST

In the years 1973-1977 an individual outpatient SST-project has been carried out at the 'Ambulatorium van het Paedologisch Instituut' in Amsterdam. Twenty-nine youths volunteered to participate. The therapist was assisted by co-therapists, students of the 'Free University' in Amsterdam. They served as an extra model for youths in real life situations (such as a pub in town, a flowershop where a youth worked, etc.). The youths had been referred by family custody associations and observation homes of the Department of Justice.

Research design

The training project included outcome research. For this purpose a therapy- and a control-group were formed, each consisting of 29 boys. The control group did not receive any training. Altogether 32 boys had been referred for training. Three of them did not accept any therapy. The groups were comparable with regard to family and living situations, and as to offences. In both cases there were 22 boys who had committed offences, varying from theft to manslaughter. The remaining 7 youths had serious behavior problems. A prognosis was made for each boy, making use of the file material available. This prognosis, the COMT-score, originates from the AEPRA-research by Brinkman and Kars (14). The prognosis for both groups was similar: more than 50% chance of failure with regard to recidivism or placement in a correctional or treatment setting. In both groups the age varied from 14 to 20 years. Age and prognosis were the main selection criteria. Drug addicts were excluded. The effects of the SST-program were determined with the aid of a questionnaire. These lists were completed by the probation officer of the youth, 6 to 8 months after termination of the training. The questionnaire comprised a large number of psychosocial variables. Additional figures were assembled regarding offences and placements in a correctional home/youth prison.

Training set-up

The social skills training sessions differed from the traditional forms of therapy on various points. The length of the therapy varied from 15 minutes to 3 hours and the frequency varied from 1 to 4 times a week. As a result of their chaotic way of life some boys occasionally did not turn up, or turned up at times other than had been agreed upon. This required a flexible time-table of the therapist and co-therapist. The training sessions were made as attractive as possible. The boy was offered a beer or snacks; the topics selected for the SST-session were selected in such a way that an optimal motivation from the youth could be expected.

Topics of the training were: association with peers and grown-ups, such as girls, bosses, and parents; learning to handle quarrels at home; mastering conflicts without becoming the underdog and without violence; looking for and keeping a job; study problems; sexuality; being able to handle money.

The techniques included: learning of new behavior with the aid of reward procedures; discrimination training (learning to differentiate between a situation in which certain behavior is relevant and situations in which it is not); self-regulation procedures; modelling and behavior rehearsals in vivo and in role-play; behavioral contracts, for instance concerning agreements between the boy and his parents; behavior counselling, etc.

What happens in such a training session? A slightly adapted description of such a session, the third session with Jan, gives an impression.

> The therapist knows that Jan has been stealing repeatedly. He is also part of a sort of 'gang' in the neighborhood of his home. He has repeated clashes with his mother's friend, who has been living with them for the last two years, and with whom he does not get on Occasionally there are rows in which physical violence is used. Jan has occasional jobs. He has many conflicts at work, leading him to leave the job or to his discharge. Apart from the gang-members he has neither friends, nor a girl-friend.
>
> During the first interview Jan was told by the therapist and the co-therapist what kind of things he could expect during the next interviews. The SST was presented as some kind of shop in which Jan could 'buy' interesting skills.
>
> In the second session Jan gave a detailed description of his daily life. On a large sheet of paper he jotted down, with a felt pen, the incidents which occurred in his daily life during a normal week. The large sheet of paper with divisions of days and hours, was pinned on to the wall. From these data and from the file the therapist knows what Jan's daily life looks like. He now also knows the names of Jan's colleagues at work, his friends in the gang, and he knows something about his preferred activities, which enables him to treat Jan more personally.
>
> Prior to the third session the therapist and the

co-therapist have made a session plan. Underlying this plan is the hypothesis that Jan's inability to associate with authority-figures at home or at work, is the basis of many problems. The conflict with mother's boy-friend leads Jan to spend a great deal of time outside the home and roaming around with his gang-friends. The conflict at work leads to discharge, which in turn leads to lack of money and roaming the streets. The plan consists of teaching Jan to handle the conflicts with figures of authority. At first, however, the therapist/co-therapist must know precisely how these conflicts take place. For this reason they will suggest that Jan acts a recent quarrel in front of the video camera. They expect the acting and the subsequent viewing of the videofilm to take up the entire session.

Jan arrives -20 minutes later than agreed upon- at the institute.

Jan: 'Yes, I'm a bit late, ain't I?'

Therapist: 'I suppose you've been very busy?'

Jan: 'Yes, I helped Theo to tune his car engine. He's going on a trip to-morrow'

Co-therapist: 'Gosh, he must be pleased. Are you so good with cars?'

In this way they talk for 5 to 10 minutes, while having a drink. Although it seems like 'small talk' the therapist and co-therapist are constantly rewarding positive behaviors with stimulating remarks, like for instance in this case the tuning of Theo's car. At the same time they are very keen on getting information which may be useful in the further training. At a given point the therapist announces the session plan as follows:

Therapist: 'Yes, Jan, I've been thinking about what we could do this evening and now I've got a proposal to make. Just tell me what you think of it. OK?' Jan nods.

'Look, last week you told me that things are not so good at home in the evenings. That your mother's friend -Piet, was his name?- is sometimes difficult if he wants to watch a different TV-channel than you do...'

Jan: 'Yes, but that's no problem. If that guy wants to be difficult I just go away to my friends...'

Therapist: 'Well exactly, that can certainly by a very good solution. But I've been thinking, and I asked myself whether Piet realizes that you are 16 years old and so quite grown-up, and that you also have your rights at home. And then I thought: perhaps that's a good subject for this evening: What do you do with someone who has no idea of your rights?'

Jan: 'Hm...'

Therapist: 'Look, I know it sounds vague at the moment, but what I want to suggest is this: you try to remember what happened during the last occasion that Piet was difficult about the TV. Then Peter (co-therapist) and I will try to act that quarrel while you are directing us. Like a play on television and you're our director. We videotape the whole thing and you operate the camera. OK?'

Jan agrees to the proposal; operating the camera especially appeals to him. While 'directing' he furnishes a lot of new information about the conflict situation. This is also part of the plan; the therapist asks him many details.

Therapist: 'You must help me a bit, otherwise I can't play Piet's role. Did he call you names? Did he hit you?' Or: 'Well, we don't have somebody around who can play your mother, but does it actually happen that your mother interferes in the quarrel?' Then the therapist and co-therapist start acting while Jan operates the camera. He can't stop laughing. Afterwards he explains the differences between the role-play and the real situation, thus supplying additional information.

> Thereafter they review parts of the videofilm. The therapist explains what was happening during the quarrel. Every now and then the picture is put on stand-still and a pose or facial expression of one of the players is pointed out, and the therapist explains what can be learnt from these. Breathlessly Jan looks at the video scenes and suddenly he asks: 'So if I want to quarrel I can cause a quarrel myself?'

We see the use of various techniques: modelling, role-play, verbal reward, stimulation of self-observation - the first phase of self-regulation. Jan's last remark, which is authentic, marks the beginning of self-observation. The video-tape made him realize that he could influence the situation around him.

Results

T-tests were carried out on a number of follow-up variables. These variables were chosen on the basis of a factor analysis of the above-mentioned follow-up questionnaire. Most of them showed significant differences in favor of the social skills training-group.

Table 1. Incidence of recidivism.

	Social skills group (n=29)	Controls (n=29)
Recidivism	7	20
No recidivism	22	9

Tables 1 and 2 show the differences in two important variables: recidivism (contacts with the police, with the exception of traffic offences) and referral to a correctional institute during the follow-up period.

Table 3 gives the means and standard deviations on six other variables on which the social skills group scored significantly ($p<.05$) better than the controls (on a five-point scale).

For a detailed account of the results the reader is referred to references 12 and 15.

Table 2. Incidence of referral to correctional institute.

	Social skills training group	Controls
Referral to a correctional institute	2	19
No referral	27	10

Table 3. Scores on six variables obtained from five-point scales. With exception of variable two, a low score means a positive judgement.

	Social skills training group		Controls	
	Mean	Standard deviation	Mean	Standard deviation
1) Serious behavior problems at home	1.37	.69	2.82	1.54
2) Number of months the youths worked during follow-up	4.86	1.84	2.75	2.54
3) Overall functioning in home or residence	2.31	1.04	3.66	1.23
4) Progress during follow-up period, as judged by probation officer	2.00	1.00	3.03	1.3
5) Association with (foster)parents	2.77	.82	3.38	.71
6) Association skills	2.29	.61	2.90	.86

CONCLUSION

The results of the project show that an outpatient social skills training can be attractive to youths in trouble. Only 3 out of 32 youths refused treatment in which participation was voluntarily. The follow-up results are promising, especially if one takes into account that this particular population normally derives little benefit from traditional forms of psychotherapy.

Following this project efforts were made to introduce the social skills training approach in different sections of the Dutch youth care system. Probation officers were trained in social skill training techniques (16) and a residential social skills training program was introduced in a state correctional institute (17,18). The development and introduction of this program is described in more detail in chapter 11 of this volume.

Note: At the 'Ambulatorium van het Paedologisch Instituut' a long-term research project (from 1973 till 1984) is carried out. The aim of the project is the development of the treatment programs for youth in trouble and their families. The researchers are: A.A.J. Bartels, J. Heiner, G. de Kruijff and N.W. Slot. Research assistents are: M.A. Berger and M. Lancee.

REFERENCES

1. Twentyman CT, Zimering RT. 1979. Behavioral training of social skills: a critical review. In: Progress in behavior modification, vol. 7. Hersen M, Eisler RM, Miller PM (eds). New York: Academic Press.
2. Bellack AS, Hersen MH. 1979. Research and practice in social skills training. New York: Plenum Press.
3. Kanfer FH. 1973. Behavior modification: an overview. In: Seventy-second yearbook of the National Society for the Study of Education. Chicago: National Society for the Study of Education.
4. Bandura A. 1969. Principles of behavior modification. New York: Holt.
5. Tharp RG, Wetzel RJ. 1969. Behavior modification in the natural environment. New York: Academic Press.
6. Kanfer FH. 1975. Self-management methods. In: Helping people change. Kanfer FH, Goldstein AP (eds). New York: Pergamon.
7. Braukmann CJ, Fixsen DL. 1975. Behavior modification with delinquents. In: Progress in behavior modification, vol. 1. Hersen M, Eisler RM, Miller PM (eds). New York: Academic Press.
8. Aiken TW, Stumphauzer JS, Veloz EV. 1979. Behavioral analysis of nondelinquent brothers in a high juvenile crime community. In: Progress in behavior therapy with delinquents. Stumphauzer JS (ed). Springfield: Thomas.
9. Junger-Tas J. 1973. Sociale integratie van jeugddelinquenten in ontwikkelingsperspectief. Nederlands Tijdschrift voor de Criminologie 15, 4-24.
10. van der Ploeg JD. 1976. Isolement, angst en agressie. Alphen aan den Rijn: Samsom.
11. Verburg A. 1981. Aan het zelfconcept gerelateerde, psychologische variabelen bij adolescenten. Doctoraal scriptie. Amsterdam, VU, Vakgroep Ontwikkelingspsychologie.
12. Bartels AAJ. In press. Outpatient social skills training for youth in trouble. Principles, results, perspectives. Lisse: Swets and Zeitlinger.
13. Phillips EL, Wolf MM, Fixsen DL, Bailey JS. 1976. The Achievement Place model: a community-based, family-style, behavior modification program for predelinquents. In: Analysis of delinquency and aggression. Ribes-Inesta E, Bandura A (eds). Hillsdale, New Jersey: Lawrence Erbbaum.
14. Brinkman W, Kars H. 1974. Aanpassing en predictie van aanpassing. Den Haag: Staatsdrukkerij.
15. Bartels AAJ, Heiner J, de Kruijff G, Slot NW. 1977. Onderzoek effecten van ambulante gedragstherapie aan 'delinquente' adolescenten (EAGDA). Amsterdam: Ambulatorium van het Paedologisch Instituut.
16. Bartels AAJ, Heiner J, de Kruijff G, Slot NW, Vogel A. 1980. Trainingsonderzoek gedragstherapie gezinsvoogden. Amsterdam: Ambulatorium van het Paedologisch Instituut.

17. Slot NW, Bartels AAJ, Heiner J, de Kruijff G, Distelbrink M. 1980. Gedragstherapie 3: een onderzoek naar het effect van het invoeren van een training in sociale vaardigheden op basis van gedragstherapeutische methoden in residentiële centra voor probleemjongeren. Eindverslag deel I en deel II (bijlagen). Amsterdam: Ambulatorium van het Paedologisch Instituut.
18. Slot NW, Heiner J, Bartels AAJ, de Kruijff G, Berger MA. 1982. Gedragstherapie 3: een onderzoek naar het effect van het invoeren van een training in sociale vaardigheden op basis van gedragstherapeutische methoden in residentiële centra voor probleemjongeren. Deel III: vervolg effectonderzoek. Amsterdam: Ambulatorium van het Paedologisch Instituut.

11. THE IMPLEMENTATION AND EVALUATION OF A RESIDENTIAL SOCIAL SKILLS TRAINING PROGRAM FOR YOUTH IN TROUBLE

N.W. SLOT

INTRODUCTION

Social skills training (SST) appears to be an attractive as well as an effective way to teach youth in trouble how they can avoid getting into trouble again and how they can manage their own life. In chapter 10 in this volume design and results of an outpatient SST are discussed. That chapter also contains the theoretical background of the SST-approach. The view taken here represents a behavioral view, in the sense that the problems of youth in trouble (adolescents having and causing problems, which brought them to the attention of the juvenile court) are seen as resulting from daily life social skill deficiencies. The residential SST-program described below is based on the same behavioral principles. The reader is referred to the previous chapter for the underlying theories.

The implementation and evaluation of the residential SST-program described in this chapter was the third project in a long-term study, from 1973 to 1984, carried out by researchers of the 'Ambulatorium van het Paedologisch Instituut' in Amsterdam (the researchers are: A.A.J. Bartels, J. Heiner, G. de Kruijff and N.W. Slot).

DEVELOPMENT OF THE PROGRAM

After the positive results of the earlier outpatient SST-program became known in the field of Dutch youth care, several institutes for youths in trouble asked for residential applications of the social skills approach. It was decided to select two institutions in which a residential SST-program should be developed. The SST-program had to be incorporated into the existing forms of treatment. In neither of the two institutions did a well-defined form of treatment exist. The researchers were faced with a dilemma: the program had to be developed within the conditions of the institutions. Therefore no standard training package could be presented to the institution telling them: 'This is the program you requested, go ahead and work with it'. On the other hand, it seemed unwise to approach the workers in an institute saying: 'We are going to look around in your institute, we will add some nice behavioral procedures here and there and we'll see where we will end up'. We decided to develop an outline for a residential SST-program before entering the institutes. This outline was meant to form the basis for the ultimate program.

The outline was derived from the Achievement Place program, a semi-residential SST-program which was also an important source of inspiration for the outpatient SST-program. Achievement Place was the name of a home in Lawrence, Kansas, U.S.A., where 8 to 10 youngsters lived together with a married couple. This couple, assisted by an alternate, made up the entire staff of the home. In Achievement Place -which was founded in 1969- the youths learned a wide range of social skills, varying from simple skills like frying an egg, and making a bed, to complex interpersonal social and community skills. The youths had jobs or went to schools in the vicinity. They were encouraged to make contacts with boys and girls in their neighborhood. Various researches (1) have shown that the Achievement Place program is effective compared to more traditional treatment settings for youth in trouble. Now there are more than 120 Achievement Place homes, which are spread all over the United States, Canada, and Mexico, and the model is also being applied in group homes for other populations including Indian youths, brain damaged youths, and drug addicts.

The Achievement Place program can be divided into three components. The outline for the residential SST-program was developed on the basis of these three components which are described below.

Token economy

Every day the youths can earn points each time they show behavior on which social skills training is focussed, the so-called 'target behaviors'. Inadequate behaviors usually lead to a loss of points. Group leaders or house parents (called teaching parents in Achievement Place homes) should be instructed to take special notice of positive behavior. At the end of the day a youth will normally end up with more points earned than lost. With this surplus, extra privileges like a free phone call, off-ground permission, the use of video cassettes can be 'bought'. The number of points lost or earned each time is written down by the youth himself on a point-card, together with a description of the behavior in question. The basic principle of a token economy, the losing and earning of points following inadequate or adequate behavior, originates from operant conditioning theory. Writing down the behavior involves aspects of cognitive behavior therapy. In terms of Kanfer's self-regulation theory (see previous chapter), the youths learn self-observation and self-evaluation.

Teaching

Group leaders or house parents teach the youths new skills by means of short behavior instructions or by demonstrating and rehearsing the skill together with the youth. Teaching can occur at any moment of the day, any time a youth shows a lack of social skills. The concept of teaching has implications for the way group leaders or house parents deal with disruptive behavior. Teaching does not simply mean suppressing disruptive behavior, but telling or showing the youth the appropriate behavior.

Semi-self government

Semi-self government means that the youths themselves participate in the development of the SST-program. They can also partly set the goals of the program, rules and consequences in the home. The longer youths have been in the program, the more responsibility they get. This system provides 'older' youths with more status, enabling them to serve as a model for new participants. Semi-self government counteracts the development of a subcultural hierarchy among the youths.

The outline, consisting of the above three components, formed the starting point for further program development.

THE CHOICE FOR THE IMPLEMENTATION OF AN SST-PROGRAM IN A TRADITIONAL INSTITUTION

Ideally, an SST-program is set up in a new home or institution. This gives the researchers the opportunity to hire new staff, to train staff members before the actual start of the program, and -if necessary- to change the physical environment. Introduction of an SST-program in a traditional institution in which a more or less defined treatment program exists, is far more difficult. In this project, however, the setting up of a new program was not possible. The Dutch Department of Justice mainly provided funds for research which could result in an improvement of existing treatment programs. This policy is quite understandable, considering the fact that during the last decade a number of institutions of the Department of Justice had got into trouble. The number of youths placed in an institution decreased dramatically during recent years. In 1967 15.024 youths lived in an institution as a result of a juvenile court decision. In 1980 this figure was 5.561. This development resulted in a reorganization which caused some institutions to merge and others to close down. In the same period of time the traditional concept of residential care became increasingly the subject of criticism. New programs which had been developed as an answer to these criticisms often failed. This situation caused the government to choose a policy of improving existing programs instead of initiating new treatment experiments.

IMPLEMENTATION AND FURTHER DEVELOPMENT OF THE RESIDENTIAL SST-PROGRAM

Implementation of a program includes: training, providing information for everyone involved with the program, negotiating with the administration about organizational changes, carrying out (interim) evaluations. Implementation can be seen as a cyclic process: in each cycle a part of the program is developed and evaluated. When it becomes clear from evaluation that a particular part of the program does not produce the expected results, this part is re-designed and evaluated again during the next cycle. This form of evaluation, during which the phenomenon under study (e.g. a treatment procedure, a production process) is further developed on the basis of feedback obtained from previous evaluation cycles, is called action research.

The implementation was started in two institutes, a home for girls with serious behavioral problems and a state correctional institute. During the initial phase of the implementation, the researchers obtained information on different aspects of life in the institution: treatment procedures, daily life routine, rules and customs in the house, attitudes towards treatment of workers and youths. The information obtained made the researchers realize that the girls' institution was on the verge of collapsing. It appeared that the administration had asked for the SST-program, hoping that this new approach would inspire a demoralized, overworked staff. After three months we decided to freeze the implementation until certain conditions -like more staff workers- were fulfilled. One-and-a-half months after this decision the administration decided to close down the institute. In this case the implementation of an SST-program resulted in a clarification of the organizational problems within the institute and precipitated the close-down.

The implementation in the state correctional institute took a different course. It was decided -after the initial phase- to start the introduction of the SST-program in one of the six cottages of the institution. Ten boys, with a staff of five, live in each cottage During the daytime the boys visit schools, vocational training centres, or the gymnasium, located on the premises of the institution. Most boys attend one or more special kinds of treatment: individual therapy, speech therapy, verbal skill training. Ironically enough, no relationship existed between the treatment goals of the special treatment and the goals in the cottage, at school, or at the vocational training centre. As a result the youths were confronted with confusing situations: they were -for example- taught during verbal skill training (with the aid of toy telephones) how to answer a telephone, while in their own cottage only staff members were allowed to use the telephone! Group leaders were in favor of the SST-program but therapists, teachers, and vocational trainers were less enthusiastic, fearing that the SST-program might interfere with their work.

The SST-program was introduced step by step. The development of a token economy took more than 6 months. Some major tasks were:

1) establishing a new organizational structure which would guarantee an effective communication between staff members of the experimental cottage, administration and researcher;
2) creating extra time for training of staff members;
3) establishing the basic conditions for research, e.g. the introduction of a daily observation log in three cottages and negotiations with the administration on matters like the random assignment of new inmates to different cottages;
4) explaining the token economy in the various areas of the institute and practising different components of the token economy with the youths themselves;
5) procuring extra rewards for the youths participating in the token economy.

Once established, the token economy functioned smoothly. Staff members, as well as the youths participating in it, described the system as a concrete and attractive way of dealing with each other. The group leaders found the system helpful in paying attention to the positive behavior of the boys Research showed positive results in the experimental cottage (see the following section). The introduction of the token economy was followed by training of group leaders in teaching techniques. A start was made with the teaching of telephone skills. The youths also learned how to wash their clothes instead of sending them to the central laundry. Individual boys learned to accept criticism in role play sessions. After one year an important part of the SST-program had been implemented in the cottage It was agreed that the program would be extended to the school and to the vocational training centre. Unfortunately, conditions deteriorated from that moment on.

The attention and support for the program from the administration became weaker due to illness and to vacancies. Group leaders of the experimental cottage felt isolated and sometimes ridiculed by their colleagues. False rumors, like the youths being rewarded for breaking the windows, spread through the institution. The four group leaders, declaring that the carrying out of the program was too much of a burden for them under these conditions, demanded a fifth group leader for the experimental cottage. The administration had to turn this demand down since all extra staff capacity had been spent on a cottage in which 3 months previously a second experiment had been started. This experiment had been set up by an administrator who was antagonistic to the SST-project. This meant the end of the SST-implementation. Sixteen months after the start in the experimental cottage the program was abolished. In the middle of these adversities one positive fact for the researchers remained: the institution cooperated in the follow-up research during the next few years. The follow-up results showed a remarkable difference between SST- and non-SST-youths (in favor of SST). These positive results make the abolition of the program even more regrettable.

EVALUATION OF THE RESIDENTIAL SST-PROGRAM

Subjects

Youths living in the experimental ('E') cottage were compared with youths in two control ('C1' and 'C2') cottages where no SST-program had been introduced. New inmates had been randomly assigned to an E-, C1- or C2-cottage from the start of the project. The youths, aged 16-19, were convicted by a juvenile court. Pre-treatment scores were obtained with the aid of an adjustment-prediction instrument: the COMT-score. This score is based on a multiple regression equation which comprises variables like: intra-family relationships, job aspirations, number of offences, behavioral disorders, neuroticism, extraversion and I.Q. All these variables are derived from available file material (2). E-youths and C1- and C2- youths did not differ on this score, which means that their psychosocial problems, reflected in the prognosis, were equal (more than 50% chance of recidivism).

Materials

Data were obtained from different sources.

1) A daily observation log completed by group leaders of the E-, C1- and C2-cottages.
2) An evaluation questionnaire regarding the behavior of the youths during their stay in the institution. Staff members from the various sections judged each boy every 12 weeks on this list. In this way we obtained several evaluations (at 12 week intervals) of the E-, C1- and C2-boys. Note that a boy's first evaluation could coincide with the second, third or even fourth evaluation of boys who had been living in the institution for a longer period. In this study we used the data of each boy's <u>first</u>, <u>second</u> and <u>last</u> evaluation.
3) A social climate scale (3) which was completed every 3 months by the E-, C1- and C2- youths themselves.

4) Interviews with E-youths during and after their participation in the SST-program.

Results

Daily observations showed that E-youths were judged better than C2-youths during their stay in the program (the data of Cl-youths were not used since the Cl daily log was not properly filled in). The observations concerned simple social skills like: getting up on time, tidying their own room, proper use of language during mealtimes. T-tests, calculated on the scores of the first 14 weeks of the SST-program, showed a significant difference on all skills observed. After 14 weeks there was no difference, with the exception of the use of proper language, on which the E-youths were judged better throughout the whole research period.

Analysis of the 12-week-evaluation of the youths showed interesting results. The evaluation questionnaire included four dimensions:

1) overall functioning (OF);
2) quality of relations with other youths in the institute (QR);
3) the number of behavior problems (BP);
4) contact with the police while on leave (CP).

E-youths were compared with Cl- and C2-youths on these 4 dimensions on their first, second and last evaluation. Figure 1 shows the results of these comparisons.

T-tests on the scores of the first evaluation showed a significant difference ($p<.05$) in just one single case (a difference between E- and Cl-youths on the dimension OF). T-tests were two-tailed because no difference between E- and Cl/C2-youths was expected after just 12 weeks of SST.

One-tailed T-tests on the scores of the second evaluation, however, showed significant differences in favor of the E-youths in 5 out of 8 comparisons. This was in accordance with our expectation. However, the comparisons on the scores of the last

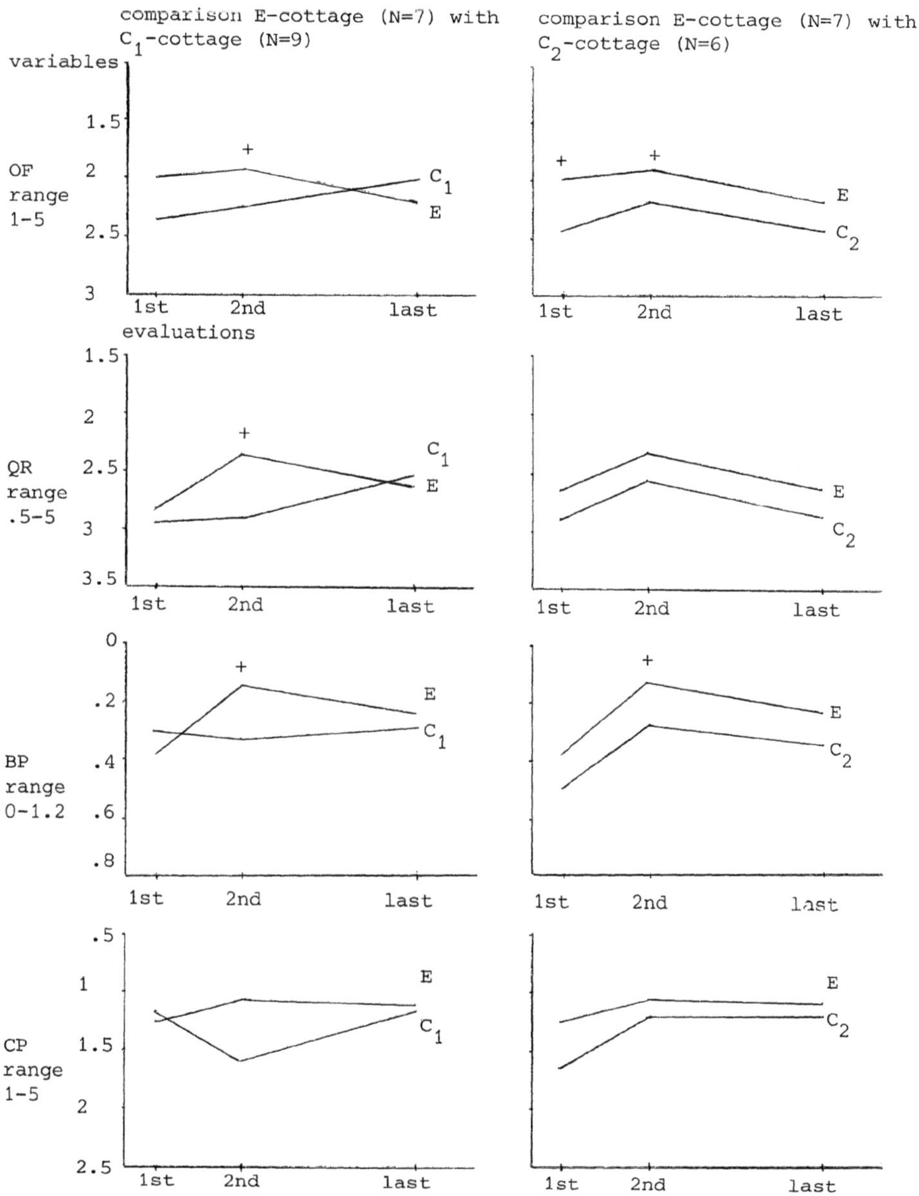

Figure 1. E-cottage evaluations on four variables compared with C1- and C2-evaluation. Lower score represents a better evaluation. Significant differences are marked with +.

evaluation show a decline for E-youths on all 4 dimensions. T-tests (one-tailed, because differences were expected) failed to show any significant results.

These results suggest that the SST-program yielded most of its effectiveness at the second evaluation, at a point of time when the youth had participated 6 months in the program. The deterioration of the E-youths after the second evaluation -though in accordance with the results of the daily observations- was not expected. Follow-up results may offer an explanation, as we will see in the following.

Comparisons of social climate data did not produce any results, with the exception of one clear finding: the social climate in the E-cottage deteriorated in the period during which the earlier mentioned organizational problems became manifest.

In interviews two weeks after the start of the SST-program the E-youths showed themselves in favor of the program (based on a set of questions offered them by the researchers; the youths had been interviewing each other). Two months after the termination of the SST-program the youths' opinions were mixed: some were still favorable, others not. Surprisingly, the youths showed themselves capable of pinpointing clearly the problems which had led to the abolition of the program.

Follow-up research showed surprising results. E-youths were compared with C1- and C2-youths on 18 follow-up variables On 16 of these variables E-youths showed better results than C1-youths. In comparison to C2-youths, the E-youths were superior on 15 variables.

On the basis of earlier research in which the same follow-up list was factor-analysed, 6 main follow-up variables can be distinguished among the 18 original variables:

1) overall improvement during follow-up period (IMP);
2) the number of contacts with the police during follow-up period (excluding contacts as a result of traffic offences) (CPOL) ;
3) the number of serious behavioral problems in the situation

where the youth lived, during the follow-up period (PROB);

4) the level of social skills in contacts with peers, teachers, employers, during the follow-up period (SKIC);
5) the number of months in which the youth had a job or attended a school during follow-up period (SJOB);
6) the difference between pre-training and follow-up COMT-score (DCOMT).

Table 1 shows the results of T-tests (one-tailed) and the differences between E- and C1/C2-youths (C1- and C2-youths are grouped together since no outstanding differences were found between C1- and C2-youths on the 18 follow-up variables). As is apparent from this table, the E-youths show better scores on all

Table 1. Comparisons of the scores on six variables between E- and C1-plus C2-youths.

Variable	N	Mean	S.D.	T-value	P-value
IMP: E	9	1.44	1.33	-2.51	.01
C1 + C2	17	3.00	1.58		
CPOL: E	9	.67	1.41	-1.05	-
C1 + C2	17	1.53	2.27		
PROB: E	9	1.44	.73	-1.43	-
C1 + C2	17	2.24	1.56		
SKIC: E	9	9.00	4.47	-2.22	.025
C1 + C2	17	14.41	6.52		
SJOB: E	8	5.38	1.60	1.80	.05
C1 + C2	15	3.67	2.41		
DCOMT: E	9	1304.00	525.36	1.05	-
C1 + C2	17	996.82	786.77		

the main follow-up variables. In three cases (IMP, SKIC and SJOB) the differences are statistically significant. The comparison on the remaining three variables (CPOL, PROB and DCOMT) does not show significant results. It should be noticed however that the results on these variables are fully in conformity with the significant findings on IMP, SKIC and SJOB.

DISCUSSION

The most striking finding in the project is that a treatment program which ultimately appeared to be successful had to be put an end to because of organizational problems. The development of an effective program seems to be simpler than bringing about the necessary organizational changes. In our opinion there is a need for applying findings from organizational change research to the field of residential treatment. In the literature on residential treatment programs one finds elucidations of treatment principles and descriptions of results, but relatively little attention is paid to the process of development and introduction of the program. An exception to this is Wetzel and Hoschouwer with their manual for program development in residential settings (4). Another salient finding in this project concerns the effects of the SST-progran on the E-youths during their stay in the institute and after they had left. As will be recalled, the effects of the SST-program were limited to the first 6 months during which the youths participated in the program. After 6 months the E-youths seemed to relapse. The question arises as to how the positive follow-up results of the E-youths after a period of 6 months can be explained if the worsening of the E-youths' evaluation during their stay in the institution signified a real deterioration? Did the lower evaluations of the E-youths at the end of their stay really represent a decline to the pre-treatment social skills level? It may be hypothesized that youths receiving training in social skills become increasingly less suitable for treatment in a traditional residential environment which, by its nature, does not give room for a large number of newly learnt social skills. In such a case the lower evaluations after 6 months could result from the fact that the youths with 'too much' social skills became a nuisance for the staff.

Our data do not permit a definite conclusion on this. We recommend further research on the implementation of SST-programs in institutions. The pressure on the organizational structure as a result of such an implementation could itself prove fruitful in bringing residential treatment closer to society.

ACKNOWLEDGEMENT

The study was financed by the Youth-care Research Committee of the Dutch Department of Justice and a private fund (Nederlands Comité Kinderpostzegels).

REFERENCES

1. Wolf MM, Phillips EL, Fixsen DL. Achievement Place: Phase II. Final report for grant nr. MH20030, from the Center for the Study of Crime and Delinquency. Rockville, Maryland: National Instititute for Mental Health. May 1, 1971 through April 30, 1974.
2. Brinkman W, Kars H. 1974. Aanpassing en predictie van aanpassing. Den Haag: Staatsdrukkerij.
3. Moos RH. 1974. Evaluating treatment environments. New York: Wiley.
4. Wetzel RJ, Hoschouwer RC. 1981. Program development and staff training in residential environments. Tucson: Intermountain Center for human development.

12. SUICIDAL BEHAVIOUR AMONG ADOLESCENTS

R.F.W. DIEKSTRA

INTRODUCTION

Suicidal behaviour among the young, perhaps even more so than among adults, has always been a distressing phenomenon both to the public and to suicidologists, as the students of suicidal acts are nowadays often called. One obvious reason is that death and suicide seem so incompatible with the idea of youth, which for many is synonymous with joy, absence of sorrow and a promising future. This apparent incompatibility has even given rise to the widespread belief, currently, and in the past, that suicide did not occur among children and adolescents.

However, throughout history, we find reports of suicide epidemics among young people, which usually are described as a matter of great concern to the community. About their causation and the way the community managed them we know little more than the often very subjective opinions of historians. The fact that they did occur, however, proves that suicide in youth is not the dubious privilege of our time or of modern civilization and its institutions, as has sometimes been suggested. When for example, in 1903, Otto Weiniger, the author of SEX AND CHARACTER (at the age of 23) put an end to his life, which appeared to instigate a wave of suicide among European high-school and university students (1), the schools became the target of public attack, and pedagogy was made the scapegoat for the self-destructive acts of young people. The first symposium on suicide, organized in 1910 by the Vienna Psychoanalytical Society and chaired by Alfred Adler, addressed itself in particular to suicide among adolescent students. In his address to the meeting Wilhelm Stekel exclaimed: 'What can be the reason for the alarming increase in

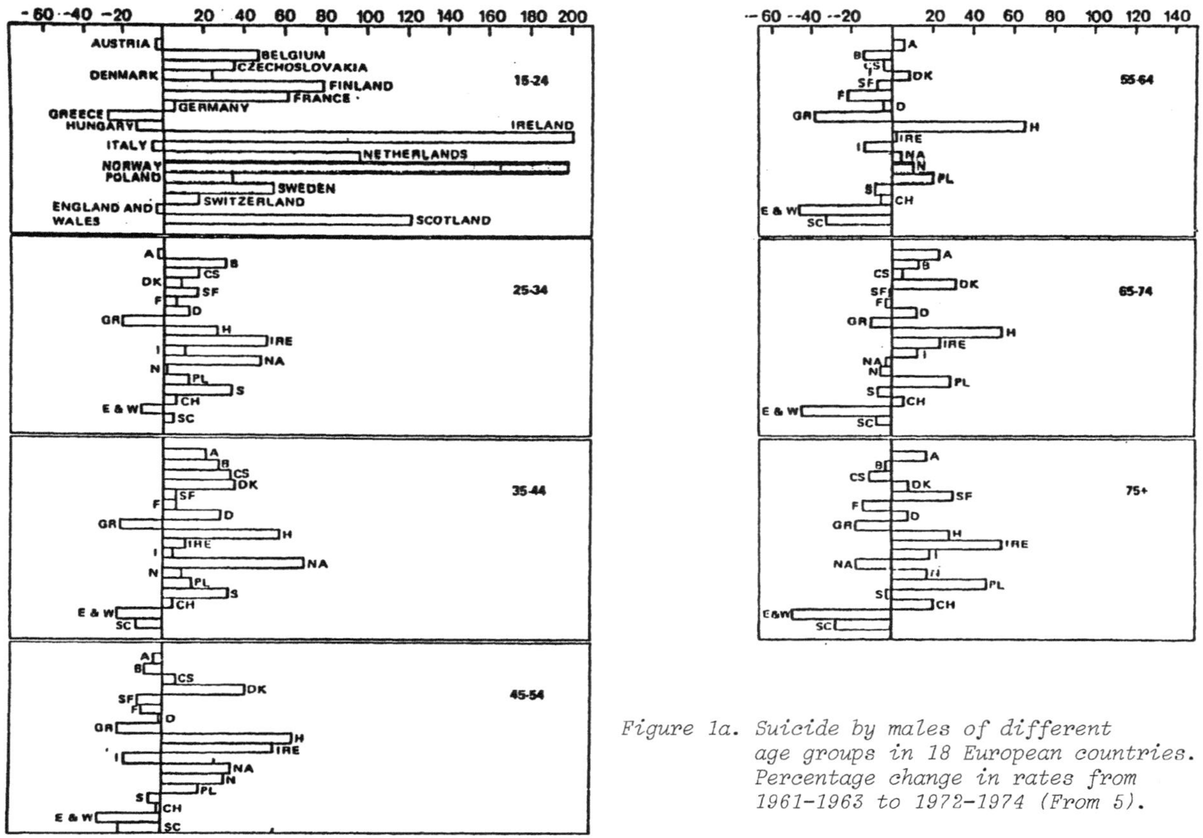

Figure 1a. *Suicide by males of different age groups in 18 European countries. Percentage change in rates from 1961-1963 to 1972-1974 (From 5).*

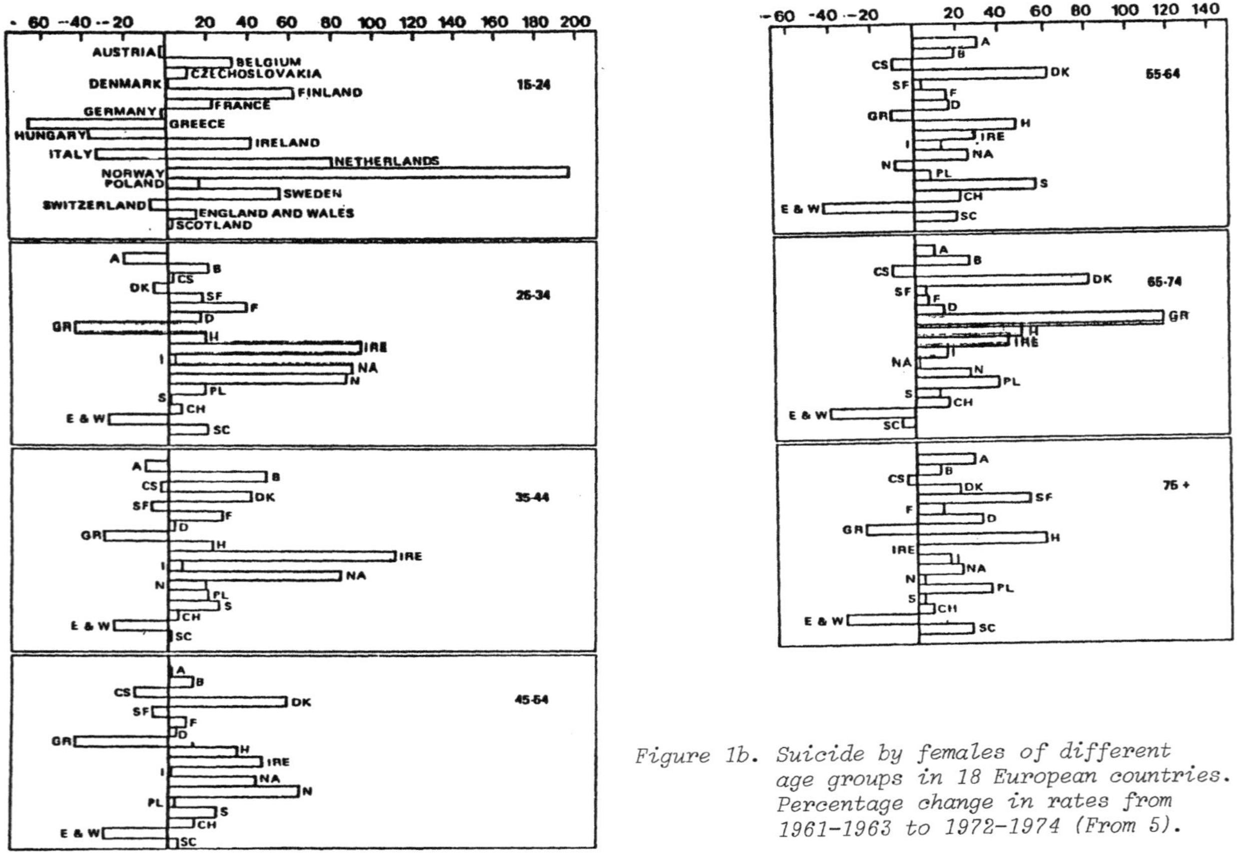

Figure 1b. Suicide by females of different age groups in 18 European countries. Percentage change in rates from 1961-1963 to 1972-1974 (From 5).

the suicide rate among young people ...?' (2). Exactly that same question is asked by modern suicidologists.

ON THE EPIDEMIOLOGY OF SUICIDE AND ATTEMPTED SUICIDE

In most countries in western Europe the suicide rate among the young has steadily increased during recent decades (see figure 1a and 1b). Also in those countries where the overall rate has decreased, or remained stable, the rate of young suicides has usually gone up. But even with increasing total rates, one can usually observe a shift in age distribution, in that the rate among the elderly remains stable or even decreases, while at the same time the rate among the younger groups rises sharply

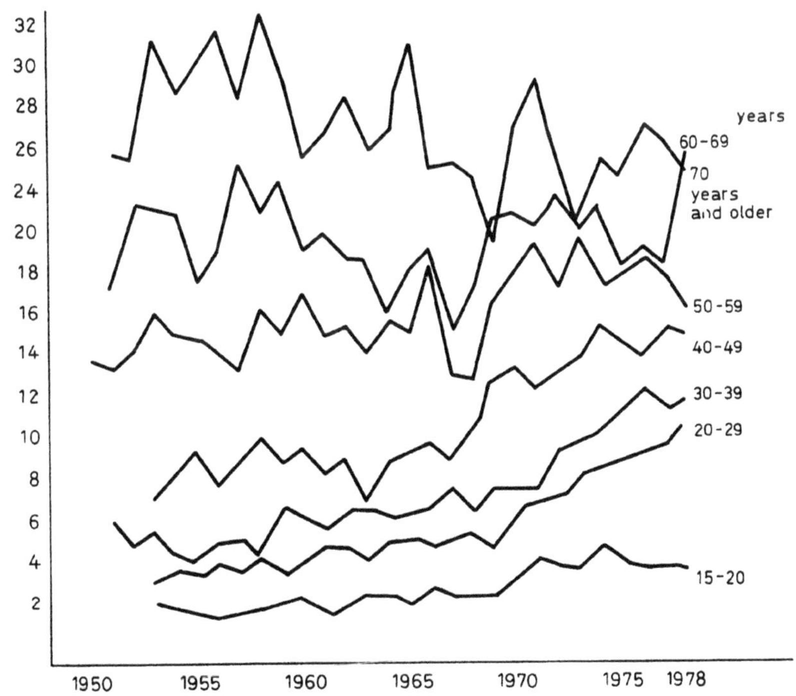

Figure 2. Suicide by age per 100.000 of population in The Netherlands (From Central Bureau of Statistics, The Netherlands).

(figure 2). According to a publication of a commission of the European Community (3), suicide ranks as the third most important cause of death in the group 15-29, causing about 10% of all deaths in the countries of the European Community. Recent research (4,5) has shown that there is no simple or definite explanation for this increase. It has become clear, however, that certain Durkheimian variables such as lack of social cohesion in a particular community, social isolation, unemployment, instability of relationships (e.g. high divorce rate), and overcrowding are, not surprisingly, related to the incidence of suicide. Some authors also suggest that the prevailing cultural attitudes of greater permissiveness towards suicide, especially among the young, plays a role (6).

From an epidemiological point of view however, the suicide trend among the young might very well be explained by another phenomenon that has spread more and more over the countries in the western world since World War II, namely that of attempted suicides, especially in the form of intentional self-poisoning. Previously, this problem seemed epidemiologically of little importance and the number of studies on attempted suicide was relatively small. Some of the first medical students of suicidal behaviour however, already pointed out that attempted suicide might involve many more people than successful suicide. For example, Esquirol (7) said in 1838: 'Of one hundred persons who attempt suicide only 40 succeed'. Nearly 20 years later, in 1856, Brière de Boismont (8) wrote that for every suicide there are two attempts. Westcott in his book SUICIDE, of 1885 (9, pp. 156-158), also paid attention to the relative importance of attempted suicide versus completed suicide, and to the uncertainty about the size of the problem when he wrote: 'As a summary of all cases reported to me, the numbers were in the relative proportion of 21 failures to 12 completed instances'. The same author seemed well aware of the possibly different meaning and etiology of attempted suicide and successful suicide: 'It is a common idea that many attempts are made with a view to coerce or influence relations and friends, attempts, which in fact are not intended to be successful although they sometimes succeed'. Generally, however, attempted suicide was seen as a by-product of suicide itself, as a bungled suicide, and consequently a phenomenon that did not require specialized study. This attitude among suicidologists gradually changed in the fifties, mainly as a result of the growing number of non-lethal suicide attempts. But also there was growing optimism that through shifting the attention away from suicide towards attempted suicide, avenues to suicide prevention would be opened. Until then progress in this direction had not been very encouraging. Gradually it became clear that in general suicides and suicide attempts form two different but overlapping populations. The significance of the overlap may be formulated as follows: someone who has once made a suicide attempt has a much higher chance to eventually die by his or her own hand. As a result, many studies are directed towards finding characteristics that distinguish high risk attempters from attempters with a low risk of successful suicide. Detection of high risk attempters would allow for specific and effective interventions that in turn might reduce the number of suicides. Such a strategy appeared increasingly necessary as the number of attempted suicides rose, and therewith the 'overflow' from this population to that of the suicides.

Studies in Great Britain were among the first that reported an alarming increase in attempted suicides. Smith (10) showed that from 1966 to 1970 hospital admissions for self-poisonings increased by 100% in Sheffield, and that in 1970 self-poisoning accounted for 10% of all medical admissions and almost 20% of medical emergencies. Based on these data, Smith estimated for Great Britain as a whole 70.000 hospital admissions per year for self-poisoning. In 1977 Jones (11), who also used data from Sheffield, estimated at least 100.000 of such admissions per year. Kreitman (12) showed that in Edinburgh from 1962 to 1974 the number of parasuicides, a term which he prefers to use instead of attempted suicides, increased by 250%, a figure also based on hospital admission data. Alderson (13) studied data from the hospital inpatient inquiry between 1953 and 1972, and he concluded that there had been a dramatic increase in the number of admissions for self-poisoning in England and Wales. Recent studies in other cities in the United Kingdom and in other countries show that this development is common to the European Economic Community (14). In The Netherlands, for example, the number of admissions to general hospitals following suicide attempts almost doubled in the period 1970-1979 (15).

The majority of suicide attempts are made by the younger age groups, that is below 35-40 years of age. Both between countries and sexes there is some variation in the peak age for making such attempts. For example in Edinburgh the modal age for women in 1976 was between 15-19, while in The Netherlands and Denmark the age curve peaks between 25-34 for women.

> A possible explanation of this difference is Kreitman's assertion (12), that classification of cases on the bases of the External cause of injury-list (E-list) of the International classification of diseases (ICD) instead of solely on the bases of the Nature of injury-list (N-list), leads to a selection of fewer and more serious cases, i.e. cases in which the intention to die is stronger. Such a selection would affect the age distribution of women more than that of men, since men generally appear to make more serious attempts and use more effective methods, while among women serious attempts occur above all in the higher age ranges. The modal age found for males and females in the studies in The Netherlands seem to support this hypothesis. The fact that the incidence rates we found in The Netherlands are considerably lower than those of the British studies also appears to be explained by this hypothesis.

In some studies the peak age for men is below, but in others above, that for women. In all studies the trend is that the rate decreases with increasing age. It is important to notice that in a 1975 general sample survey in The Netherlands the age distribution appeared not to be different from that of the other studies, namely peak ages between 15 and 24 and decreasing rates for age groups 25 and older (16).

In view of the fact that the phenomenon of attempted suicide has grown to epidemic proportions in the last 20 years, and that it is particularly characteristic of the young, along with the overlap between attempted suicide and suicide, one can predict that the suicide rate among the young will rise to a degree that will be reflected in national mortality statistics. The question as to what causes the increase in suicide has to be formulated as: what causes the increase in attempted suicides?

Despite the increasing number of studies and the growing epidemiological, psychiatric and psychological knowledge on suicide attempters, this question has not yet been satisfactorily answered. Many of these studies give divergent or even contradictory results, probably as a result of the different socio-economic groups and areas that have been studied. The implication is that there are probably different types of suicide attempters and of suicide attempts, and therefore both theory and research should be directed towards building a valid and useful typology. On the other hand it is also important to examine what is common to all the different types of suicide attempters. Most relevant in this respect seems a recent study by Braucht (17) in Denver, Colorado, the results of which indicated that mutual interactions between particular kinds of individuals, their environments, and the occurrence of specific stressful events -what could be thought of as mismatches between individuals and their ecological niches- are systematically related to the desire to end life itself. This is an other way of saying that attempted suicide is a behaviour characteristic of minority sections of the society as a whole or of specific regions, towns, districts or neighbourhoods. Unemployment, race, sex, age, poverty, social isolation, or a combination of these, could give rise to specific forms of incongruence with the environment. In his book SUICIDES (18), the French author Baechler stated that suicide attempts are often characteristic of groups or individuals who are dependent for their well-being on other more powerful institutions or persons, and that attempting suicide is often the only, or at least one of the few, acts that mobilizes one or other of them into some response. Such a position of relative powerlessness or dependency, given the infrastructure of our societies, is to a high degree characteristic of groups like women, the unemployed, and the young!

A TYPOLOGY OF SUICIDAL BEHAVIOUR

Like adults, adolescents show all the possible varieties of suicidal behaviour, lethal and non-lethal suicide attempts, and suicidal ideation. Compared to the older age groups, however, the suicide rate among adolescents, although significantly increased over recent decades, is both relatively and absolutely low. Furthermore, if we consider all kinds of suicidal behaviour, it is to be noted that suicidal acts among the young have a fatal outcome much less often than among older groups. To try to understand this it is helpful to look at suicidal behaviour from a social learning point of view (19). From this perspective behaviour in general can be regarded as having two sorts of outcome: <u>direct</u> and <u>indirect</u>. For example, if I hold a loaded gun against my head and pull the trigger the <u>direct</u> effects of that behaviour will be brain tissue damage, loss of consciousness, and probably biological death. <u>Indirect</u> effects involve the reactions of other persons to my behaviour, such as their efforts to stop me, to save my life, to care for me, to mourn over my decease etc.

Generally speaking, if we select a behaviour we do this because we expect to attain a goal, or solve a problem, as a direct, indirect or both direct and indirect, effect of that behaviour. The extent to which the direct or indirect effects of suicidal behaviour are expected to be effective is likely to be related to the lethality of its outcome. If the expectancy of effectiveness of the direct effects is very high, as far as the solution of problems is concerned, and the expectancy of effectiveness of the indirect effects (i.e. reactions of others) is at the same time very low, the probability that the behaviour has a lethal outcome is very high (real suicide). Vice versa, if the expectancy of direct effects is very low while the expectancy of indirect effects is very high, the probability that the behaviour has a non-fatal outcome will be very high (manipulative suicide attempt). If we give the sum of these expectancies the value of one, we can formulate the relationship between both expectancies as a continuum in which we can distinguish three major positions, namely:

1. $E_d : E_i = 1 : 0$
2. $E_d : E_i = .5 : .5$
3. $E_d : E_i = 0 : 1$

The three ratios correspond with the three main categories of suicidal behaviour, namely 1) the (real) suicides or suicide-attempts with an almost certain lethal outcome, 2) suicidal attempts with an uncertain or ambiguous outcome (the bulk of suicide attempts), and finally 3), suicide attempts with an almost certain non-lethal outcome (the manipulative attempt) where the medical seriousness is low, or very low.

It is important to consider the factors on which the ratio E_d/E_i depends, of which two main ones will be mentioned here. The first is the degree of irreversibility of the disruption the suicidal person is confronted with. For example, a terminal illness is a situation that cannot be escaped from as a result of the indirect effects of a suicidal act, but only by its direct effects. Therefore, suicide attempts under such circumstances have a high probability of a lethal outcome. On the other hand, failure to pass an exam is often not an irreversible situation, so that a suicide attempt for such a reason will rarely end in the death of the actor.

A second important factor lies in the effects experienced in previous suicide attempts. For example, if a previous suicide attempt, in which the medical seriousness was low, only resulted in antagonizing significant others, and worsening relationships with them, the E_i will probably decrease while the E_d may rise, so that a subsequent attempt may easily be fatal. Since disruptions in the early stages of the life cycle, such as adolescence, are relatively seldom irreversible, it would follow logically from the previous reasoning, that the E_i of suicidal acts should on the whole be relatively high, and the probability of a lethal outcome relatively low. Accordingly, we would predict relatively more non-lethal attempts among the young than among older people, and relatively less suicides, which is exactly what is observed throughout the western world. However, since previous attempts can change the E_d/E_i ratio when their expected indirect effects did not occur, groups that show an increase in suicide attempts, such as adolescents do, will probably also show an increase in actual suicides, a prediction that is borne out by the data we have presented in the first part of this paper. There are two corrollaries we can derive from our reasoning. Firstly, since expectancies of behavioural consequencies have to be learned, either by observation or by practice, an important factor in a theory of suicidal behaviour should be the suicidal behaviour repertoire of an individual. Logically, suicidal acts cannot be sufficiently explained by the types of disruption or problems a person has to cope with. The fact that somebody suffers a loss, or the fact that somebody suffers from a mental illness, such as schizophrenia or depression, is not a sufficient explanation of why he or she attempted or committed suicide.

From a review of the literature on the relationship between depression and suicidal behaviour, Diekstra (20) draws the conclusion: 'Summarizing, depression has proved to be an important condition in the genesis of suicidal behavior in a great many cases. However, since not all suicidal persons are depressed and not all depressed persons suicidal, a depressive illness cannot legitimately be seen as the necessary and sufficient condition for suicidal behavior'. The same applies to the relationship between suicidal behaviour and other psychopathological syndromes. There can be no doubt that mental illness plays an important role in the process that leads to suicide or suicide attempts in many cases, but again not all suicidal persons are mentally ill, and suicide itself cannot be considered an indication of mental illness. Besides, suicidal behaviour or suicidal tendencies are not dependent upon, or derived from, any clinical entity found in present day psychiatric nosology. This means that efforts to classify suicidal persons according to available diagnostic categories is often a hazardous enterprise. Several authors (21) also include alcoholism and drug addiction within such a scheme, whereas strictly speaking both terms refer to behaviours, not to specific syndromes with a specific etiology. However, not only these, but also a number of other behaviours have frequently been proved to be antecedents of suicidal behaviour, which brings up the issue of behavioural correlates of suicidal acts.

BEHAVIOURAL CORRELATES OF SUICIDAL ACTS

Diekstra (19) tested the hypothesis that neither antecedent events or problems, nor personality characteristics (as measured by standard psychological tests), but rather behaviour repertoire characteristics would be the most powerful predictors of attempted suicide as the reason for admission to a general hospital. In a study based on 580 admissions of which 109 following a suicide attempt, the hypothesis was supported in that the most powerful predictors were (in the following order): 1) previous suicide attempt(s); 2) previous threats of suicide or suicidal ideation; 3) alcohol, psychopharmaca or hard drug abuse; and 4) suicide, or suicide attempt(s), or behaviour equivalent to suicidal behaviour among significant others. Personality characteristics and life events, or so-called precipitating events, also explained some of the variance, but less than the behavioural indices, and only in interaction with them.

These findings are relevant for a number of reasons. First of all because they show that the occurrence of attempted suicide, being a behaviour and not a disease entity, in the presence of conditions that predispose towards such behaviour (such as depression), depends upon the suicidal behaviour repertoire of a specific individual. Thus, whether suicidal behaviour will occur under such conditions, depends upon the availability of suicidal or related acts within an individual's behaviour repertoire, or, in simple terms, on the extent to which the individual has learned to act suicidally in these circumstances. This has been nicely demonstrated by the data from Barraclough and Pallis's study (22) comparing depressives who committed suicide with others who did not. The depressed suicides had made a suicide attempt ten times more often than the living depressives (41% versus 4%)!

There are various ways in which individuals can learn to react with suicidal acts under specific conditions. First of all there is the possibility of direct learning (previous suicidal gestures or attempts by the person himself). Secondly, vicarious or observational learning can have taken place, as for example, by observing how a significant other attempts or commits suicide while being depressed or on encountering a severe personal loss. Kreitman et al. (23) demonstrated that suicidal behaviour was significantly more frequent among significant others of suicidal persons than in a representative sample of the general population. Diekstra and van Gestel (4) replicated this study and were able to demonstrate that the influence of suicidal models was very specific. <u>Suicide attempters did not have significantly more significant others who committed suicide, but had indeed more significant others who attempted suicide!</u>
This might explain why the incidence of attempted suicides or parasuicides has increased enormously over the last decades in most European countries, while at the same time the incidence of actual suicides has remained stable or even decreased.

From a behavioural point of view it is also not surprising that drug addiction or toxicomania, either on the part of the person himself or of significant others, is predictive of suicidal behaviour. For most suicidal acts are performed by using poisonous substances. In a way most suicidal acts can be considered to be a form of abuse of drugs. Once a person is accustomed to the use of drugs, the intake of an overdose (which then is defined as a suicide attempt or a suicide) is often just a matter of time.

The same applies more or less to alcohol abuse. Those who chronically and excessively drink alcohol usually have, either as a result of their drinking or for some other reason, severe personal and social problems. Once they have taken to coping with these problems through the intake of a mind changing chemical substance (i.e. alcohol) the use of other chemical substances in high doses (such as psychopharmaca) also becomes highly probable. Not surprisingly, the incidence of suicide among alcohol abusers is high, about 15% (24). The same applies to the incidence of alcohol abuse among suicide attempters (15-30%, 19). The percentage of suicides among drug (predominantly opiate) addicts is estimated to be about 10% (24).

The increase in suicide and attempted suicide among adolescents over recent decades might at least be partly explained by changes in their pattern of drug abuse, since it has been shown, for example (25), that the proportion of suicide attempts among women in Edinburgh aged 15-24 years following consumption of alcohol, doubled between 1968 and 1974. Also, in those countries where an increase in admissions for attempted suicides has been reported, a dramatic increase in alcohol consumption among the young has been observed during the same period (20). Some authors suggest that the increase in attempted suicides might largely be a consequence of more liberal prescribing of psychotropic drugs by doctors. The proportion of self-poisonings by prescribed versus non-prescribed drugs, however, has hardly changed since 1962, which makes this explanation rather improbable.

ADOLESCENCE: FIRST ENCOUNTER WITH DEATH

The late Erwin Stengel (26) once made the statement that at some time in his evolution man must have discovered that he could do away with his life, since when his existence has never been the same. When in the life history of mankind this might have happened Stengel did not say, although he mentioned the awakening of consciousness or self-consciousness as a marking point. If we assume that the evolution of mankind in general repeats itself more or less in the life cycle of each individual, a hypothesis that has been made by many giants in the field of science, then the question arises concerning the stage in the life of the individual when he or she usually begins to consider or think about possibility of suicide.

Several studies (6) show that the majority of people never seriously harbour the thought of suicide or think about the possibility of committing it. Although there is some variation in the estimates, a maximum of 25% of samples of the general population that have been investigated admit to having had such thoughts. These 25% seem to differ in two important ways from the rest of the samples. Either they are better educated or they more often have a history of long-standing problems, or both.

The greater education among those who had thought of suicide is something that already in 1922 was mentioned by Bayet (27) in his momentous work LE SUICIDE ET LA MORALE, in which he gives a historical overview of the development of western moral views concerning suicide. Bayet made a distinction between what he called a 'morale simple' and a 'morale nuancée'. 'Morale simple' refers to an absolutely negative and prohibitive view of suicide, which has a pagan origin. He held that it has always been typical of the lower social classes, the uneducated and the ignorant. The 'morale nuancée' refers to a relatively permissive attitude, according to which suicide is considered acceptable or excusable under certain circumstances. It has usually been the attitude of the aristocracy and the intellectual or educated classes.

In this part of the 20th century in the western world higher education has become more common than ever before in history, especially among the younger age groups (below 40-45), who were born after World War II. Not surprisingly then, the studies referred to above show, that the age at which suicide begins to be considered seriously, is adolescence, covering the developmental stage between 12 and 21 years of age. Indeed, already as early as twelve years some children begin to consider suicide seriously (28). Usually these children are above average in intelligence and in life experience.

The fact that it is in adolescence when thinking about suicide appears for the first time, is of significance in itself. It is customary to define adolescence as that stage in life when the transition from childhood to adulthood has to take place. In primitive cultures this transition was often symbolized by or embedded in special initiation rituals. For example, the youngster might be completely wrapped up in clothes like a cocoon and put in a cabin where he or she stayed for several days without anything to eat or drink. Then a special ceremony would take place during which the youngster was gradually unwrapped like a butterfly emerging from its cocoon and was then dressed like an adult. The ritual clearly symbolizes that the child has to die before the adult can be born, and expresses the idea that adolescence is the period in life when for the first time the human being has the task of consciously developing a relationship with death, whether as something to be feared most of all, or as a possible option under certain circumstances, such as by suicide.

Indeed, before the age of twelve suicide is a very rare event, but thereafter it becomes of increasing importance as a cause of death. This is not only true in our time, but was probably true of all cultures at all times in human history. However, today suicide is becoming more and more important, and more and more common, at an earlier stage of the human life cycle, and the question arises as to how we are to explain this trend. Can it be attributed to the better education of the young, or do the problems of living, largely of a social character, have a more important influence than formerly?

SOCIAL FACTORS IN ADOLESCENT SUICIDE

It is widely established that suicide and attempted suicide are associated with a variety of social problems including criminality, unemployment, interpersonal difficulties, and childhood separations. The associations of these variables with suicidal behaviour are particularly strong among the younger age groups and have shown no change over the years (29). Boor (30) found that over a period of 14 years in a number of countries in the western world the association between the unemployment rate and the suicide rate is especially strong among the young. Rutter (29) points out that the prevalence of social problems in the community in general has been rising, and that it may well be that in part the increasing attempted suicide rate reflects the increasing presence of these social stressors. Diekstra and Kerkhof (31) provide further evidence that social stressors might affect young people more deeply than the elderly, to the point of eliciting suicidal tendencies. In a factor-analysis on the answers to a suicide attitude scale taken from two samples of the general population they found two main factors that could be interpreted as follows:

1. respondent's ability to imagine any circumstances at all in which he/she, or others, might commit suicide;
2. estimated probability of physical and social problems as reasons for committing suicide by respondent or others.

Relevant for the present discussion is the fact that on the second factor there was a significant difference between the age groups in factor scores. The older and younger groups hardly differed in estimated probability of suicide in situations like incurable or terminal physical illness or chronic psychiatric disturbance. They did, however, differ very significantly in estimated probability of suicide under adverse social conditions, such as loss of job, or breaking off of a relationship etc. The younger age groups considered the probability that they or others would commit suicide under such circumstances much higher than did the older age groups. Apparently, the longer people live, the better they are in general able to cope with the social vicissitudes of life, and conversely, young people seem to be more vulnerable to adverse social events.

The implication would be that the earlier in the life cycle a human being is confronted with social problems or the thwarting of future perspectives, the more psychologically disruptive will be the long term effect. When such eventualities occur in adolescence, a stage in life when for the first time a conscious attitude towards life and death has to be developed, the chances are likely to be high that this attitude will be inimical towards life and more positive towards an escape from it, in the form of suicidal or similar behaviours.

The present economic crisis with its accompanying massive unemployment and lack of social perspectives, especially for the young, makes this dreadful possibility only too realistic. A youngster who makes a suicide attempt in reaction to the unfavourable socio-economic situation he finds himself in, can seldom be helped by such practical measures as being offered a job, career opportunities etc. Little can therefore be expected in the way of constructive reactions by others, as indirect consequences of the suicidal attempt. Consequently the number of lethal suicidal acts among the young will continue to increase in the near future. In my opinion herein lies the highest priority for suicidology, namely to help to prevent the option of suicide appearing as a desirable one so early in the life cycle of the individual -as in adolescence- that life itself hardly gets any chance. This will require not so much further development of clinical strategies and skills, but rather political and social action and diplomacy in order to draw the attention of the decision makers in society to this problem.

REFERENCES

1. Szittya E. 1925. Selbstmoerder. Leipzig: Weller.
2. Steel W. 1910 In: Ueber den Selbstmord insbesondere den Schueler-Selbstmord Diskussionen des Wiener Psychoanalytischen Vereins. Wiesbaden: Bergmann.
3. Commission of European Community. 1979. Social indicators for the European Community 1960-1978. Brussels.
4. Diekstra RFW, van Gestel H. 1980. Correlaten van suicidaal gedrag. Leiden: Department of Clinical Psychology, internal report.
5. Sainsbury P, Jenkins J, Baert EE. 1981. Suicide trends in Europe. Chichester: Medical Research Council.
6. Diekstra RFW. 1981. Over suicide. Alphen aan den Rijn: Samsom.
7. Esquirol E. 1838. Des maladies mentales. Paris: Baillière.
8. Brière de Boismont A. 1856. Du suicide et de la folie suicide. Paris: Baillière.
9. Westcott WW. 1885. Suicide. London: Lewis.
10. Smith J. 1972. Self-poisoning with drugs: a worsening situation. British Medical Journal iv, 157-159.
11. Jones DIR. 1977. Self poisoning with drugs: the past 20 years in Sheffield. British Medical Journal i, 28-29.
12. Kreitman N. 1977. Parasuicide. London: Wiley.
13. Alderson MR. 1974. Self-poisoning - what is the future? Lancet i, 1040-1043.
14. Diekstra RFW. 1982. On the epidemiology of attempted suicide in the EEC. In: New trends in suicide prevention. Wilmotte J, Mendlewicz J (eds). Basel: Karger, Bibliotheca Psychiatrica no. 162.
15. Diekstra RFW, de Graaf AC, van Egmond M (submitted). On the epidemiology of attempted suicide: a sample survey among general practitioners. Crisis (Journal of the international association for suicide prevention).
16. Diekstra RFW, van Egmond M, Kerkhof A. Suicidal behavior among the general population: the results of two sample survey studies. Paper presented to the American association for suicidology, New York, 1982.
17. Braucht GN. 1979. Interactional analysis of suicidal behavior. Journal of Consulting Clinical Psychology 47, 653-669.
18. Baechler J. 1979. Suicides. Oxford: Blackwell.
19. Diekstra RFW. 1973. Crisis en gedragskeuze. Amsterdam: Swets and Zeitlinger.
20. Diekstra RFW. Psychological and psychopathological factors of suicidal behavior. Paper presented to the WHO-conference: Changing trends in suicide behaviour in Europe, Athens, 1981.
21. Lester D. 1972. Why people kill themselves. Springfield, Illinois: Thomas.
22. Barraclough BM, Pallis DJ. 1975. Depression followed by suicide: a comparison of depressed suicides with living depressives. Psychological Medicine 5, 55-61.

23. Kreitman N, Smith P, Tan ES. 1970. Attempted suicide as language, an empirical study. British Journal of Psychiatry 116, 465-473.
24. Miles CP. 1977. Conditions predisposing to suicide: a review. The Journal of Nervous and Mental Diseases 164, 231-244.
25. Holding TA, Buglass D, Duffy JC, Kreitman N. 1977. Parasuicide in Edinburgh - a seven year review 1968-1974. British Journal of Psychiatry 130, 534-543.
26. Stengel E. 1964. Suicide and attempted suicide. Baltimore: Penguin Books.
27. Bayet A. 1922. Le suicide et la morale. Paris: Felix Alcan.
28. Mack JE, Hickler H. 1981. Vivienne: the life and suicide of an adolescent girl. Boston: Little, Brown.
29. Rutter M. 1980. Changing youth in a changing society. Cambridge, Massachusetts: Harvard University Press.
30. Boor M. 1980. Relationships between unemployment rules and suicide rates in eight countries, 1962-1976. Psychological Reports 47, 1095-1101.
31. Diekstra RFW, Kerkhof A. 1982. Attitudes towards suicide in the general population. Leiden: Department of Clinical Psychology, internal report.

13. HOW ARE WE TO DEAL WITH ADOLESCENTS AND THEIR PROBLEMS?

J. DE WIT

In this summary report, I will discuss some implications of a developmental viewpoint for prevention and intervention. This implies that it is not only our task to bring all that has been said into some coherent perspective, but also to discuss the relations between descriptions (empirical findings) and possible prescriptions (intervention methods). What can we learn from these descriptions and what do they imply as regards the interventions that are needed? The question is a persisting one, and the answers can only be tentative.

During this conference we discussed and reviewed many characteristics of adolescence. There is indeed a variety of features which marks adolescence as a period of development, which to some extent differs from both earlier and later stages. Adolescence implies the conclusion of childhood and the initiation of adult life (de Levita, chapter 2 in this volume). It is a period of transition. However, there are various ways in which this transition can take place. Dasberg aptly discussed (chapter 1 in this volume) the many varieties of adolescence. Adolescence is a complex phenomenon during which we can see all kinds of interactions between developmental time, social time and historical time (1). Yet at times it still seems to be thought of in terms of the stereotype of the storm and stress concept. Also, our contemporary research is usually confined to easily available groups of adolescents i.e. nice middle class males, which undoubtedly gives a one-sided, not to say a distorted picture. I will not summarize again all the changes and characteristics of adolescence. This has already been done by Hindley (chapter 3 in this volume). Yet the question remains is there a concept that has enough integrative power to give a comprehensive and intelligible view on this period. In my view the concept of identity (2), with its corollaries of experimentation and shifting of identifications, is one which has the potentialities of applying across different cultures because it holds that developmental changes are determined by a multiplicative interaction of two sources of development: nature and nurture. It needs, however, to be operationalized in a satisfactory way, to be freed of its elitist connotations.

IMPORTANT FACTORS IN NORMAL ADOLESCENT DEVELOPMENT

Adolescence is not a break. It is not inherently a period of psychological disturbances or social alienation. Indeed if one considers all the physical, psychological, and social changes that occur during adolescence, one might expect more disturbances than actually occur. In fact, during adolescence we find many positive strengths and many abilities to cope with difficult situations. I therefore want to underline the positive factors that are to be seen during adolescence.

Firstly, I want to stress the point that during adolescence many new capacities emerge and existing capacities increase. This is quite clear in the cognitive field. Cognitive skills are becoming more powerful because of a higher level of abstraction and more flexibility in reasoning. The same can be said with respect to social and emotional skills. New powers of love and friendship emerge. We also see new differentiations in feelings towards others and more reflections on these feelings. It is clear that these changes do not develop spontaneously, but have to be learned and experienced in interaction with other people. Adolescence is very much a period during which a variety of new skills have to be learned. This implies, for example, the learning of a social grammar of courtship and lovemaking (Straver, chapter 8 in this volume). Here the hypothesis, suggested by Slot and his colleagues (chapters 10 and 11 in this volume), that delinquent behaviour can be conceptualized as due to inadequate social skills, is a very intriguing one. The adolescents in Slot's study found it revealing to experience that their behaviour always leads to consequences. It is still more revealing to learn that by altering your behaviour you can also alter the consequences, i.e. the interactions with other people. Although perhaps the youngsters we call delinquents have special difficulties in these respects, this kind of approach should not be restricted to this particular group. All of us have to learn, relearn and unlearn constantly. And the last is most difficult. In this regard I would like to underline that the conceptualizations of social learning theories as they have been developed over the last ten years provide us with many fruitful applications in the field of adolescence.

Secondly, all changes do not take place at the same time. Adolescence is a period that has been substantially prolonged during the last decades - at least in our culture. One of the positive side-effects of this rather long period of re-orientation could be that the various life crises do not coincide. Having a first love affair, often with a negative outcome -we don't have empirical findings!-; having a critical school examination; trying to enter the labour-market; these are all potentially stressful situations. Fortunately there are many school examinations and many love affairs. So each one is not at all necessarily decisive, and fortunately they seldom all occur at the same time. Therefore the adolescent can profit from what he or she has experienced before.

As we have learned from stress research, it is not simply stressful events as such, but the cumulation of stresses at the same time which is most disadvantageous. It appears that even with chronic family stresses children are not especially at risk, if there is only a single source of stress on its own. On the other hand, stresses potentiate each other, so that a combination of stresses has effects that are much more than a summation of the effects of separate stresses on their own (3). Here I would like to refer to van Seters's presentation (chapter 7 in this volume). Divorce is certainly a situation which is likely to be disturbing to adolescents. Expecially during a period when they are entering into the new field of partner-relations, the perception of models that are not very successful will certainly produce a stressful situation. But other positive and negative factors have to be taken into consideration as well.

A third observation refers to what I would like to call the life-span perspective. Defining adolescence as the period of transition from childhood into adulthood could imply that adulthood, with its capacity to love and to work, would be considered as an absolute, ideal norm. We should realize, however, that not only are there many varieties of adult life, but also that adulthood itself is a period of transition with respect to the whole life-span. During the life-span one continuously has to integrate the past and to prepare for the future. Life is a dynamic process. What does this imply for adolescence?

My conclusion is that not only do we have to look at the discontinuities in development, but also at the continuities, as for example the style of coping mechanisms which an individual develops during his life time. Neither should we make too sharp distinctions between the various periods. Sometimes I have the feeling that the prolongation of compulsory education keeps the adolescent in a rather dependent position and has a negative effect on his or her introduction to the labour-market and the world of adult life. The boundaries between school and work are much too rigid, and the extension of the period of being at school can produce many problems of adaptation to the usually invisible adult work situation. These are modern discontinuities in cultural conditioning, resulting in too sharp boundaries between the various periods of the life-span.

The fourth observation is about male and female development. I am very pleased that many findings and ideas about male and female development have been presented during this conference.

We badly need them. Adolescent psychology in its present state is still too much oriented towards male development. There is much to discuss here. What I have learned is that males are much more vulnerable than females -it is a reassuring thought to be an underdog- and that the most natural condition is the female one. It is important to recognize that boys and girls are indeed different and that these differences find their expression on several levels. However, all these findings -sometimes tentative- are difficult to interpret. We know that boys in certain respects are more aggressive than girls. There is also some evidence from ethological observations on subhuman primates that these differences in aggression are not limited to the human species. But we need to be cautious in our interpretations. Certainly, as enlightened people, we all adhere to an interactionist viewpoint, but I fully agree with Wolff (chapter 4 in this volume) that lip-service is not enough. We need to know more, indeed a great deal more, about the mechanisms that are involved in this interaction process.

Nevertheless it is valuable to know of psychological characteristics that are related to male and female development respectively. Here, I refer to Everaerd's presentation (chapter 9 in this volume): sociosexual contacts between boys and girls are guided by egalitarian concepts, but there are still traditional role expectations with regard to duty-sharing in marriage, and to sexual initiatives. The crucial question concerns which role-patterns are changing along with changes in the culture, and which are relatively stable? There is room here for a good deal of speculation, but also -I hope- for a great deal of empirical research yet to be done.

DEVELOPMENTAL DISTURBANCES

Following these observations on normal development, I would like to make a few remarks on disorders occurring during adolescence. I agree with Rutter's view (3) that although the storm and stress concept is a considerable distortion of the usual course of development, nevertheless for many youngsters the transition from childhood to adulthood is marked by an upsurge in depressive feelings, an uncertainty about the future, and an increased risk of psychological disorder. Delinquency, drug abuse as well as depressive conditions, become much more common during adolescence. However, the overall frequency of psychological disturbances during adolescence appears not to differ greatly from those of childhood and adulthood, according to the scarce epidemiological findings which are available. Furthermore there are changes in the sex ratios of incidence. For example, in childhood several types of disorders are much more common in boys, in adolescence the ratio becomes equal.

One conclusion from all these findings is that we should not conclude from a storm and stress view that emotional disturbances in adolescence are just a natural phenomenon and will spontaneously pass away. We should take them as seriously as we would do during other periods of life.

Some findings presented in the paper of Diekstra (chapter 12 in this volume) reminded me of the important distinction Rutter makes (3) between two types of disorders in adolescence: the chronic conditions, the old or persistent disorders as he calls them, and the new ones, the disorders that start during adolescence. It is quite interesting to note that the persistent disorders have strong associations with educational retardation and with many indices of family psychopathology; however, it is much more difficult to relate the new ones to particular environmental factors. These findings deserve further exploration and research in order to be more successful in the field of prevention and treatment of problems that arise during adolescence. Some preliminary research done at our institute (4) suggests that this distinction also has relevance with respect to therapy. When treated by traditional psychotherapy these new disorders have a better prognosis if intervention starts early.

IMPLICATIONS FOR PRACTITIONERS

What does all this mean for daily life, i.e. for the way practitioners deal with adolescents? Do we get a clearer picture of the normative adolescent from all these findings? Does this picture affect our expectations of the likely response of adolescents to treatment? The proof of the pudding is in the eating and therefore I invite you to play a game that has been developed at the adolescence-unit of the Paedological Institute. Here are two lists of symptoms, presented by an imaginary family doctor, who refers to a boy aged 15 and a man aged 30 years. Please read them carefully and make your assessment.

Boy, aged 15, lives with parents	Man, aged 30, married
Information:	Information:
1. dresses untidily (shabby)	1. is dressed untidily
2. refuses to do domestic tasks	2. doesn't bother with housekeeping
3. visits his grandmother every week; communicates very well with her	3. visits his mother every week; communicates very well with her
4. the only things he produces are model-boats	4. is very occupied with his model-train
5. thinks about leaving school	5. is always talking about changing work
6. but doesn't know what to become (profession)	6. but doesn't know what to do then
7. recently he has a girl-friend	7. recently he has a girl-friend
8. recently troubled with headache	8. recently troubled with headache

Now let me ask you two questions. 1) Who is more disturbed - the man or the boy? I see, that as I guessed, the majority vote is for the adult as the more disturbed. 2) Whom would we refer first for treatment? My conclusion is -and I see it is in line with your opinions- that, although the man is perhaps much more disturbed than the boy, the boy should have treatment first. What is the reason for this paradox?

My guess is that we prefer to help the boy, because he is still in development, which implies that we believe that he, being an adolescent, has more capacities to cope with his problems and to alter his life-style. Perhaps this is the essence of combining developmental findings with clinical hunches about accessibility to treatment. We believe that in this transitional stage there are many possibilities that we can stimulate. Therefore we prefer to help the adolescent boy first.

PRINCIPLES OF ADOLESCENT TREATMENT

What does adolescent treatment imply? Are there some 'golden rules'? Perhaps I may give some indications, introducing a kind of slogan, that has been developed at our institute. Treatment of adolescents should be: concrete, flexible and oriented towards future (see also: 5). What does this mean?

Concrete: this refers to the possibility to learn from new experiences in daily life. It refers to experimentation with alternative life-styles and profiting thereby. A therapist of adolescents should consider this learning in relation to real life events as an essential part of his therapy.

Flexible: this means that there are rapid changes during development and that therefore we should not be too rigid in our therapeutic activities. We must recognize that there are many changes, simply occurring spontaneously during adolescence, for which we need to be prepared. Don't be too much disappointed therefore, when adolescents change not because of your therapeutic interventions, but just because of some unforeseen events. People can also change on their own!

Orientation towards the future is a very important element in our 'slogan'. It does not refer to some remote ideal like that of a happy and healthy adult personality, but rather to the next steps to be taken in order to reduce the problems. Short-term therapies have a strong appeal in this regard because the therapist tries to define together with the adolescent, what is the first problem to solve. Usually the choice is of a relatively easy problem. Solving some problems gives rise to a very important learning experience which, hopefully, provides the possibility of transferring a problem-solving approach to other situations (6).

Time is too short to elaborate further on these points.

Certainly, therapy with adolescents is much more complicated than I may have implied in my suggestions of a 'philosophy' of treatment of adolescents. Nevertheless, I think these principles are relevant throughout the whole therapeutic spectrum from the more insight-oriented to the more action-oriented therapies.

INTERVENTIONS AND PREVENTIVE ACTIVITIES

Centering this discussion on therapeutic activities we should not forget, however, that therapy is just a small part of all the interventions and preventive activities that are possible and needed. Here we may distinguish the following areas (7).

1. Preventive policies directed at the individual predisposition.
2. Prevention through influences on opportunity and situation.
3. Ecological interventions.
4. Therapeutic interventions.

I will refer briefly to each of these in turn.

Although in nearly all cases strict scientific evidence is lacking with respect to the efficiency of well-known measures and policies, there is reasonably good evidence that there are several risk situations (e.g. poor quality of parenting) which should be reduced. However, a society without risk situations does not and never will exist. The most essential thing is to provide children and adolescents with strengths to counter the stresses and disadvantages with which they have to cope in growing up.

Our tolerant society permits rather easy accessibility to many harmful drugs (including alcohol). How can we find an appropriate response to aggression and its derivatives? We know, for example, that vandalism will occur much more easily in neighbourhoods where maintenance of buildings etc. is poor. Actions are necessary to reduce the probability of producing this kind of risk situation. It requires an active mental health policy, and as part of our mental health responsibility we must concentrate our thinking on the central question: how can we attain a society that engenders among the younger generation the feeling that it is worth living in.

Ecological interventions have too often been neglected in the past. There are many possible fields of intervention but I will restrict myself here to underlining the importance of good schools. Schools can give the adolescent much support. Teachers are important models who directly shape, one way or another, the behaviour of many individual children. However, recent research (8) suggests that schools have an overall ecological effect which goes far beyond the consequences of particular teacher behaviour on individual children. A fair response to an individual child will have an effect on the rest of the class. Therefore consistency of school values, and the establishment of some principles and guidelines, which are clearly recognizable and accepted by the school as a whole, are very important. Differences in outcome between schools appear to be systematically related to their characteristics as social institutions, and not primarily with such physical factors as the size of the school or the age of the building, nor with special educational methods. Unfortunately education and mental health are often considered to be two different worlds. We need to recognize that closer interaction and cooperation between these fields is a necessary prerequisite for more successful work with adolescents.

I have already made some remarks about treatment. Let me close by suggesting that in our therapeutic efforts we should give particular attention to how we can help those adolescents who are traditionally regarded as difficult to help because of their 'lack of motivation'. Perhaps we should recognize instead our lack of therapeutic skills with them. We are only at the beginning of learning how to deal with adolescents and their problems.

REFERENCES

1. Elder GH. 1980. Adolescence in historical perspective. In: Handbook of adolescent psychology. Adelson J (ed). New York: Wiley, pp. 3-46.
2. Erikson EH. 1968. Identity, youth and crises. New York: Norton.
3. Rutter M. 1979. Protective factors in children: responses to stress and disadvantage. In: Primary prevention of psychopathology, vol. 3: Social competence in children. Kent MW, Rolf JE (eds). New Hampshire: The University Press of New England, pp. 49-74.
4. Anbeek M, Bartels AAJ. In press. Evaluation of outpatient psychotherapy of adolescents with psychoneurotic and psychosocial problems. Child and adolescent.
5. De Wit J, van der Veer G. 1979. Psychologie van de adolescentie. Nijkerk: Callenbach.
6. Dekker A, Schraa K. 1979. Over kort gesproken. In: Psychologen over het kind, vol. 5. De Wit J, Bolle H, van Meel JM (eds). Groningen: Wolters Noordhoff, pp. 133-160.
7. Rutter M. 1980. Changing youth in a changing society. Cambridge: Harvard University Press.
8. Rutter M, Maughan B, Mortimore P, Ouston J, Smith A. 1979. Fifteen thousand hours secondary schools and their effects on children. London: Open Books.

14. EPIDEMIOLOGY AND THE ROLE OF PUBLIC HEALTH ORGANIZATIONS

F. WAFELBAKKER

The concept 'public health' has not been precisely defined, but the following characteristics may be mentioned:

- directed towards the community at large,
- strong emphasis on prevention,
- an actively anticipatory policy,
- programming from an epidemiological point of view,
- considerable government responsibility with regard to policy concerning planning, coordination and quality control.

Of these five I will refer mainly to the fourth, the epidemiological.

The demarcation of public health is also difficult, notably in relation to social welfare. Particularly as regards adolescence, these areas overlap quite clearly: if there is no employment, if there is insufficient housing for young people, if minority groups are not cared for, then well-being is in immediate danger and health is threatened.

EPIDEMIOLOGICAL ASPECTS OF ADOLESCENCE

Mortality

Measured by the death rate, the 10-14 year age group is the golden age (boys 31, girls 21 per 100.000). After this age period a relatively large increase occurs, above all as the result of accidents, especially on the road (boys 78, girls 31 per 100.000). Figure 1 shows the leading causes of death. In the ages 15-19 accidents rank first, malignant neoplasms second, congenital malformations third. Suicide, and in some countries

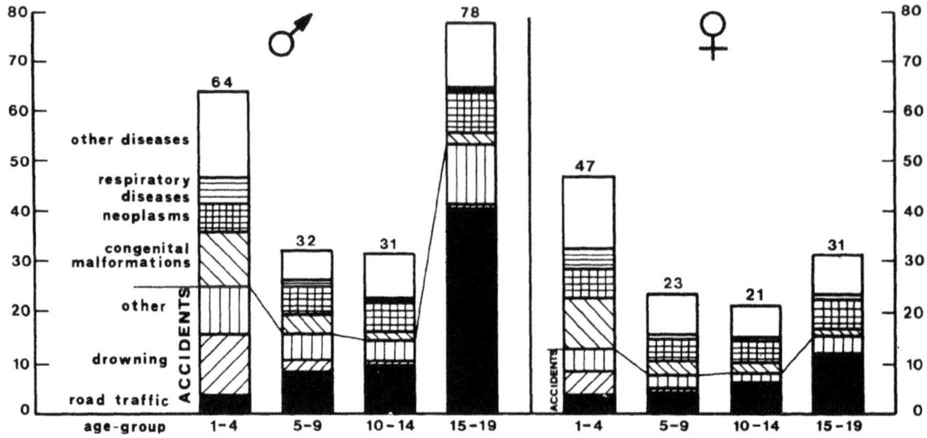

Figure 1. Causes of death in children by age and sex, per 100.000, 1979 (from 1).

homicide, ranks fourth.

International comparative research into the leading causes of death, as indicated in figure 2, is a further public health task

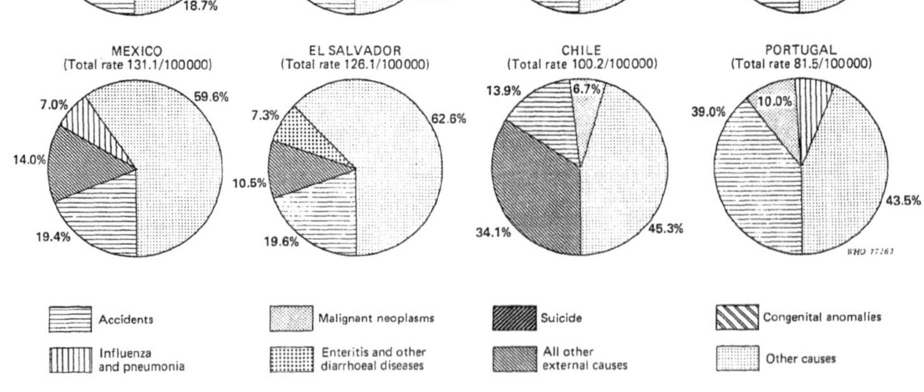

Figure 2. Relative importance of the eight leading causes of death in the age group 10-19 years, in eight countries, 1973 (from 2).

Table 1. Major health problems among adolescents.

gynaecological problems	
birth control	.contraception .morning-after pill .abortion
venereal diseases	
eating disorders	.obesity .undernutrition .anorexia nervosa
acne	
mononucleosis infectiosa	
epilepsy	
diabetes	
allergies	.hayfever .asthma .atopic dermatitis
accidents	
suicide, homicide	
drugs, alcohol	

(2). The differences between the importance of accidents and in the reporting of suicide are remarkable in these figures, which are no longer up-to-date.

Morbidity

Morbidity data have to be gathered from hospitals, outpatient clinics, school health services, surveys among general practitioners, etc. The measurement problems are difficult. There is an increasing need for epidemiological research on the health problems of adolescents. In table 1 some of the major health problems among adolescents are indicated.

MAJOR HEALTH PROBLEMS AMONG ADOLESCENTS

I will restrict myself to some of these health problems and hazards, which I approach and comment on from a public health point of view.

Birth control

Contraception

Birth control is not only a topic for men, women, and general practitioners, but also for legislators, sick funds, political parties, public health institutions and the medical inspectorate, and to various public organizations such as the Dutch organization for sexual reform and the Rutgersstichting (a family planning organization). Although general practitioners are increasingly prepared to provide very young girls with the means of contraception, a considerable number of youngsters prefer to visit one of the consultancy bureaus of the Rutgersstichting. They fear that general practitioners' confidentiality in relation to their parents is insufficiently guaranteed. Figures are available on the use of the contraceptive pill, the morning-after pill, and on abortion.

Among youngsters, aged 15-19, there is still a small increase in use of the oral contraceptive pill (table 2). In all other age groups there is a decrease. No figures are available on the use of other contraceptive methods by youngsters. However, requests for the morning-after pill and abortion provide data on failures in contraception.

For 11 years the Sentinel station project has flourished (3,4). Here, 60 general practitioners submit a weekly return on which certain illnesses and occurrences are reported. In 1972

Table 2. Percentage of women using oral contraceptives, by age. The Netherlands 1975-1980 (from 5).

	Age (y)				
Year	15-19	20-29	30-39	40-49	15-49
1975	22.3	50.4	40.2	19.4	35.6
1976	19.6	52.0	39.9	20.1	35.8
1977	18.9	55.1	38.2	19.7	36.2
1978	25.3	50.7	34.8	17.7	34.4
1979	26.6	46.2	27.6	16.1	30.8
1980	24.6	44.9	20.3	11.7	27.0

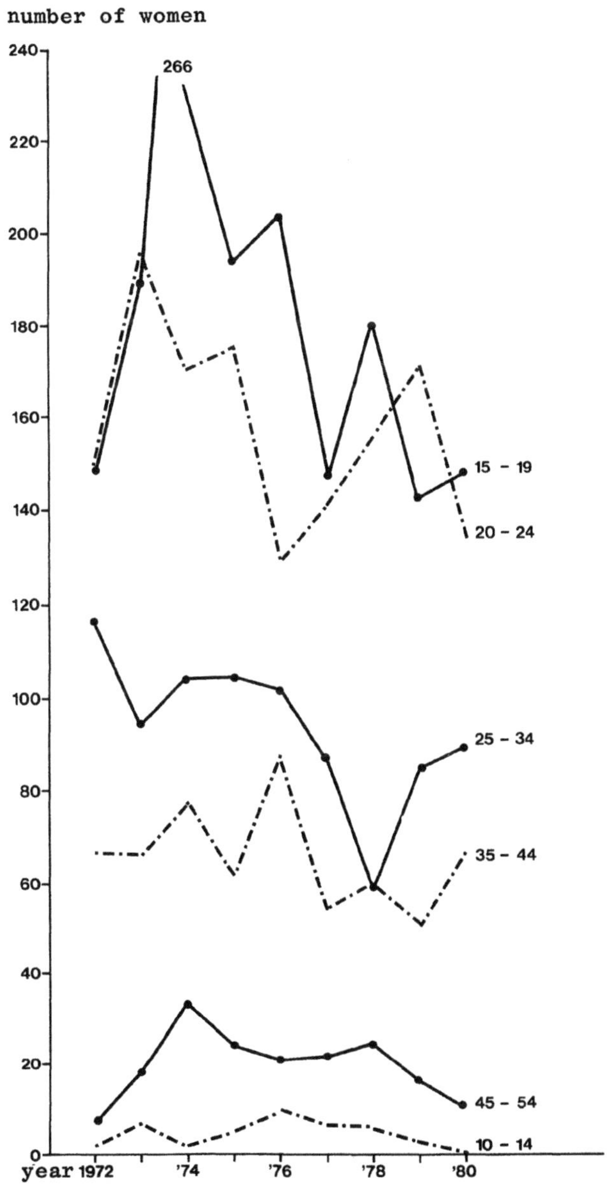

Figure 3. Prescription of the morning-after pill by age, per 100.000 women, 1972-1980 (from 4).

Table 3. Abortion, age-specific rates per 1000 women. The Netherlands 1974 and 1980 (from 5).

Age (y)	1974	1980	change in %
15-19	5.5	5.3	- 4
20-24	7.9	8.6	+ 8
25-29	6.2	7.6	+ 23
30-34	6.6	6.6	----
35-39	3.3	2.7	- 18
total	5.4	5.5	+ 2
	N=17.500	N=19.700	

the 'spotter' physicians were asked for the first time to report when they prescribed the morning-after pill (figure 3). The 15 to 19-year-old girls show the highest level in almost all the years.

Abortion

The permanent register of abortion in The Netherlands by the organizations Stimezo (6) and CBS (Central Bureau of Statistics) shows that, in the age group 15-19 years, abortion occurred in 5.3 per 1000 Dutch women in 1980 (table 3).In 1981, 52 girls of 14 years or younger had an abortion (table 4). Can we draw any conclusions? Fifteen out of 1000 girls ask for the morning-after pill and 5 out of 1000 girls have abortions, amounting altogether to 20 per 1000. Should there be an attempt, by means of health education, to diminish this remaining 20 per 1000 also? Or should one accept that Wishful Exposure to Unwanted Pregnancy (WEUP) will always lead to a number of unwanted pregnancies?

Venereal diseases

Since 1976 an obligation exists in The Netherlands to anonymously notify cases of gonorrhoea and syphilis. It is to be

Table 4. Abortion by age of women. The Netherlands 1981 (from 6).

Age (y)	n	%
≤14	52	0.3
15-19	2.652	16.5
20-24	4.185	26.1
25-29	3.486	21.8
30-34	2.998	18.7
35-39	1.876	11.7
40-44	687	4.3
≥45	90	0.5
?	92	-
Total	16.118	100.0

expected that not all cases are in fact reported, as both illnesses can progress (almost) without symptoms. In addition, the need to report is often forgotten by general practitioners. Although the peak incidence is between the ages of 20 and 30, we find already quite a number of cases between the ages of 15 and 19 years.

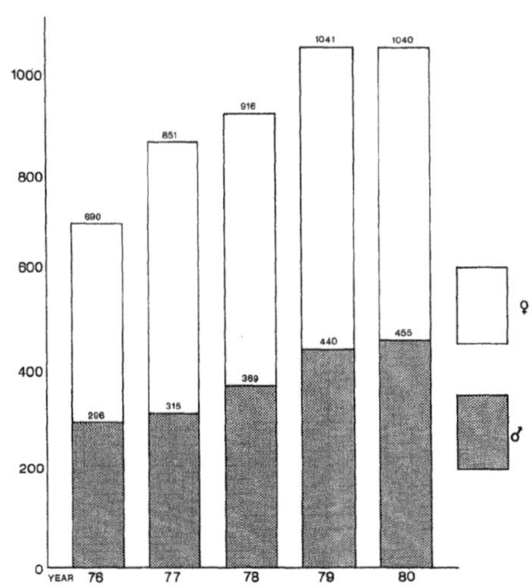

Figure 4. Notified cases of gonorrhoea in 15 to 19-year-olds. The Netherlands 1976-1980 (from 7).

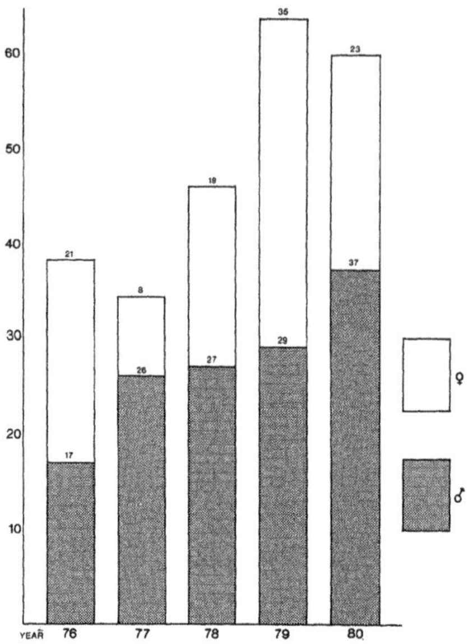

Figure 5. Notified cases of syphilis in 15 to 19-year-olds. The Netherlands 1976-1980 (from 7).

Figure 4 shows the increasing incidence of gonorrhoea. Below the age of 20 the number of girls is higher, over 20 years, boys predominate. The incidence of syphilis is also showing a gradual increase, both in the age group 15-19 years (figure 5) and in the older age groups.

The public health answers to venereal diseases are:

1. improved information, by means of methods which were not used previously, such as venereal disease telephone services and posters in railway stations;
2. better aiming at specific target groups. A number of researches show a substantial incidence of venereal diseases among homosexuals. The tracing of this group, as well as the provision of information to its members, must be very active and far-reaching, for instance by the availability of a social nurse for consultation in a homosauna, homo-bar, in brothels etc. (8);
3. among homosexuals in the helping professions (general practitioners, nurses, health educators), initiatives are

taken to remove obstacles in the medical services, especially in relation to venereal diseases.

Eating disorders

Obesity

Criteria for obesity vary and are culturally determined. We consider those 20 per cent above the mean as obese. By this criterion about 10 per cent of children in primary education, and 10 to 15 per cent of adolescents, are obese. In a few school health services experiments are being done by having group-sessions of obese adolescent girls.

Undernutrition

The recent interest in alternative and macrobiotic foods and food-habits has led some adolescents to devise their own food regimens. Some of these regimens are better than what they would ordinarily eat, but others are inadequate (9).

Anorexia nervosa

Anorexia nervosa remains obscure in its precise course. At Maastricht University inquiries are being made into the possibilities of screening-procedures in school health-services.

Infectious mononucleosis

Thanks to the Sentinel Station project (3) we have got a better insight into the incidence of mononucleosis infectiosa (Pfeiffer's disease, glandular fever, figure 6). This is a disease which is caused by the Epstein-Barr virus, which is conveyed by oral contact with exchange of saliva or droplet infection. Confirmation of the clinical diagnosis of mononucleosis infectiosa depended on a positive Paul-Bunnell

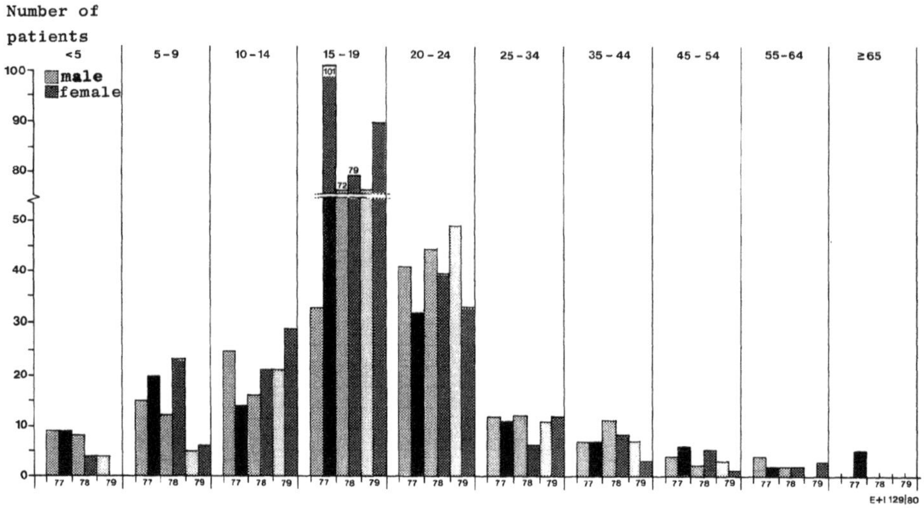

Figure 6. Mononucleosis infectiosa, by sex and age group, per 10.000. The Netherlands 1977-1979 (from 3).

reaction, a positive monosticon reaction, or a characteristic blood picture. The incidence reaches its climax in the age group 15-19 years, with girls predominating over boys (figure 6). The condition is sometimes called 'kissing disease' and the data are consistent with this name. After the age of 20 years the incidence decreases. Two possible explanations appear likely: lifelong immunity and less promiscuous kissing?

Accidents

Accidents not only constitute the main cause of death in adolescents, but the sequelae to them, in the form of long-term disability, are very costly both in human and in economic terms. A valuable source of information is the annual booklet 'Accident Facts', published by the National Safety Council in the United States. There are relevant data on school accidents, traffic accidents, and work accidents.

Table 5. School and college accidents. Deaths by age group, per 100.000 population, in 1977 (from 10).

Age (y)	Rate
1- 4	27.3
5- 9	16.9
10-14	17.7
15-19	60.1
20-24	65.1

School and college accidents

School and college accidents show a sharp rise for teenagers aged 15 to 19 years, and for youths aged 20 to 24 years (table 5).

Traffic accidents

There were about 143 million drivers in the United States in 1979. Ten per cent of them were under 20 years of age. These 14 million drivers were responsible for 5.3 million accidents. Thus 38 per cent of drivers under 20 were involved in an accident in one year. The percentages of speeding violations in fatal accidents decreased steadily from 44 per cent for drivers aged 15-19 to about 9 per cent for drivers 75 and over (table 6). However, right of way violation increased from 13 per cent for 15 to 19-year-old drivers to 50 per cent for those 75 and over.

Work accidents

All age groups of workers are most likely to suffer an occupational injury or illness during their first month on the job, but for workers less than 16 years of age, nearly 50 per cent of the reported injuries or illnesses occurred during the first month (table 7).

The incidence of injury or illness decreases with length of service in all age groups. We could call this the innovation effect. The younger the worker, the stronger this

Table 6. Category of improper driving by age of driver. Fatal accidents, U.S.A. 1975 (from 11).

Kind of violation	Age (y) 15-19	20-24	25-34	35-44	45-54	55-64	65-74	≥75
Speed too fast	44	42	40	35	29	24	13	9
Right of way	13	12	14	17	22	27	40	50
Other violation	43	46	46	48	49	49	47	41
	100	100	100	100	100	100	100	100%

innovation effect.

It is to be noted that there is a clear sex difference in the data summarized in the last three tables. The risks for boys are three or four times greater than for girls. This raises the question as to how far public health can offer any answer to the very obvious accident-proneness that young male adolescents show. Do we have to accept that some kind of selection exists within the adolescents that tends to Darwin's ' survival of the fittest'? Should we alter the age, at which a driver's licence can be obtained? Should we make it higher, or even lower? In relation to traffic accidents, one can think of training parks, but what is to be done regarding work accidents, which cause such serious damage and suffering among the youngest age groups in the first month of employment?

Table 7. Work injuries and illnesses in per cent of cases per month, by length of service and age. North Carolina and Iowa 1977 (from 12).

Age (y)	Length of service 1 month	2-3 months	4-6 months	7-12 months	2-3 years
<16	47	14	2	1	-
16-20	31	14	3	2	1
21-25	14	9	5	1	1
26-35	8	5	3	2	1

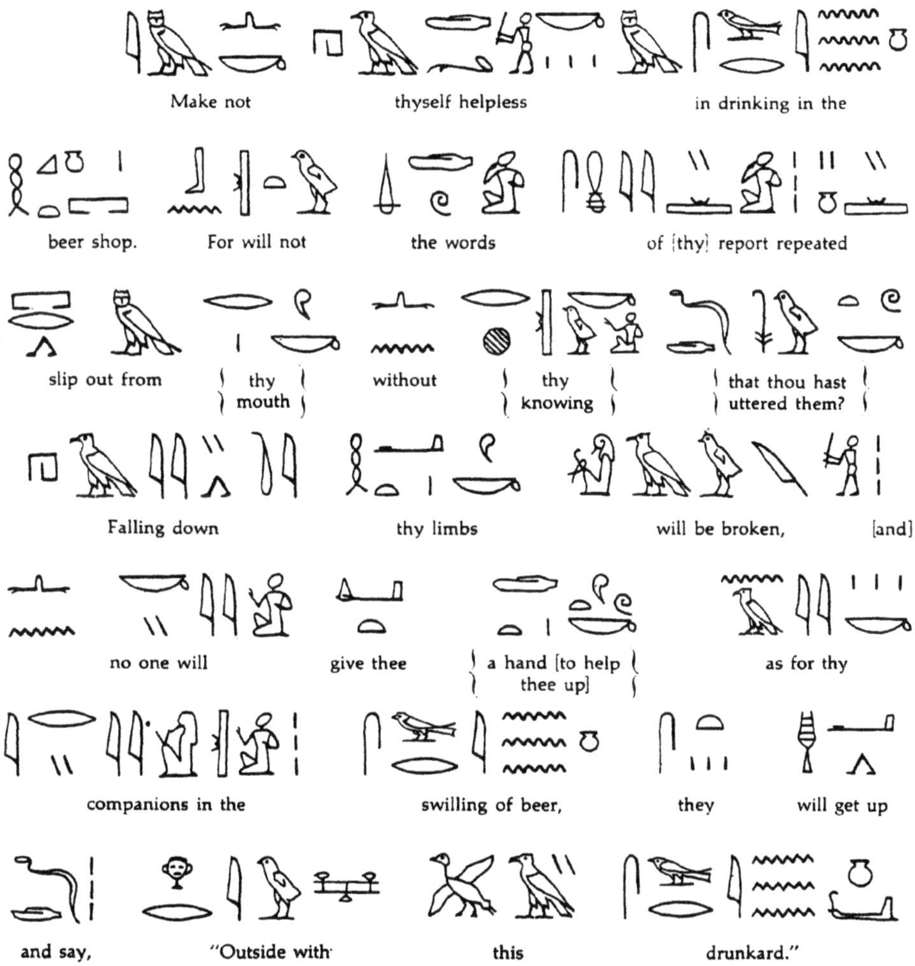

Figure 7. Cautionary remarks from an Egyptian book of etiquette. The Percepts of Ani, 1500 B.C. (from Sir E.A. Wallis Budge, The Dwellers on the Nile (from 13).

Is health education a way? The idea is a very obvious one, but we may well expect it to have little effect. Books and information on health and safety are generally rather dull. Can we not make them much more attractive? Health education also plays an important role in relation to smoking habits, alcohol and drugs. Here, experience suggests that teenagers may be more effective teachers of their peers than are adults. Programmes begun by youths themselves have proved highly effective in drug education, reducing drug abuse among youthful clients beyond all expectations. Models developed for youth-tutoring-youth programmes are also highly effective. The problem of healthy and temperate living is perhaps as old as mankind. The Egyptians at least did know how to give their advice in a very convincing way. 'Make not thyself helpless in drinking in the beershop. For will not the words of thy report repeated slip out from thy mouth without thy knowing that thou hast uttered them? Falling down, thy limbs will be broken, and no one will give thee a hand to help thee up. As for thy companions in the swilling of beer, they will get up and say, 'Outside with this drunkard'.' (Figure 7).

RECOMMENDATIONS

1. For adolescents the schooldoctor should be available for consultation at a fixed time, every week, in the school; is very desirable.
2. In addition to the usual skills the adolescent's doctor should have knowledge and proficiency in the fields of contraception and venereal diseases, with interpersonal problems, and with such personality problems as sexual identity and suicide.
3. Health education should search for approaches that are attractive for youngsters, and this should be done in close co-operation with them. Among these should be health education by peers, in the form of youth-tutoring-youth programmes.

REFERENCES

1. van der Meeren WBJM, Verbrugge HP. 1981. Youth health care in the Netherlands, 0-19 years. Leidschendam: Ministry of Health and Environmental Protection.
2. W.H.O. Expert Committee. 1977. Health needs of adolescents. Technical Report Series 609. Geneva: WHO.
3. Continuous Morbidity Registration, Sentinel Station, The Netherlands. 1979. Leidschendam: Ministry of Public Health and Environment.
4. Continuous Morbidity Registration, Sentinel Station, The Netherlands. 1980. Leidschendam: Ministry of Public Health and Environment.
5. Ketting E. 1981. De teloorgang van 'de pil'. Zeist: NISSO.
6. Ketting E. 1982. De permanente registratie abortus Nederland. Verslag over het jaar 1981. Den Haag: Stimezo.
7. Bijkerk H. 1982. Epidemiologie. In: Seksueel overdraagbare aandoeningen. Stolz E, Suurmond D. Alphen aan den Rijn: Stafleu.
8. Bleeker A, Coutinho RA, Bakker-Kok J, Tio D, de Koning SAJ. 1981. Prevalence of syphilis and hepatitis B among homosexual men visiting two saunas in Amsterdam. British Journal of Venereal Diseases 57, 196-199.
9. Frankle RT, Heusenstamm FK. 1974. Food zealotry and youth: new dilemma's for professionals. American Journal of Public Health 64, 11-18.
10. Accident Facts. 1980. Chicago: National Safety Council.
11. Accident Facts. 1977. Chicago: National Safety Council.
12. Accident Facts. 1979. Chicago: National Safety Council.
13. Katchadourian H. 1977. The biology of adolescence. San Francisco: Freeman.

SUBJECT INDEX

www.ingramcontent.com/pod-product-compliance
Ingram Content Group UK Ltd.
Pitfield, Milton Keynes, MK11 3LW, UK
UKHW020136160926
475607UK00003B/71

* 9 7 8 0 8 9 8 3 8 5 8 1 6 *